NURSING RESEARCH FOR NURSING PRACTICE

Karyn Holm, R.N., Ph.D.

Associate Professor, College of Nursing
University of Illinois
Clinical Chief, Medical-Surgical Nursing
University of Illinois Hospital and Clinics
Chicago, Illinois

Jane Gentry Llewellyn, R.N., D.N.Sc.

Associate Professor
Rush University College of Nursing
Assistant Chairperson
Department of Operating Room and Surgical Nursing
Rush—Presbyterian—St. Luke's Medical Center
Chicago, Illinois

W. B. Saunders Company 1986

Philadelphia London Toronto Mexico City
Rio de Janeiro Sydney Tokyo Hong Kong

W. B. Saunders Company: West Washington Square
Philadelphia, PA 19105

Library of Congress Cataloging-in-Publication Data

Holm, Karyn.

Nursing research for nursing practice.

1. Nursing—Research. 2. Medicine, Clinical. I. Llewellyn, Jane Gentry. II. Title.
[DNLM: 1. Nursing. 2. Research. WY 20.5 H747n]

RT81.5.H66 1986 610.73 85–19642

ISBN 0–7216–1178–8

Editor: Dudley Kay
Developmental Editor: Alan Sorkowitz
Designer: Bill Donnelly
Production Manager: Laura Tarves
Manuscript Editor: Mark Coyle
Illustration Coordinator: Peg Shaw

Nursing Research for Nursing Practice ISBN 0–7216–1178–8

Last digit is the print number: 9 8 7 6 5 4 3 2

Preface

The current escalation of knowledge mandates that practitioners be armed with the most current information. As professionals, nurses must be committed to lifelong learning both within and outside of formal educational structures. Since the basic goal of research is to uncover new knowledge, the professional who is able to evaluate, discriminate, and use current research findings will be the one who is at the forefront. Thus learning the skills of the researcher is imperative for leadership in clinical practice.

We believe that for nursing to build a scientific base, all nurses should know something about research. We do not mean to imply that all nurses should be researchers; rather, we support the notion that nurses in varying professional roles should contribute to bridging the gap between practice and research. Only then can a scientific base for nursing practice evolve and allow us to stand toe-to-toe with other professional disciplines.

This book has a threefold purpose: (1) to provide the reader with an understanding of the research process, (2) to provide a rationale for determining the relevance of a study for clinical practice, and (3) to highlight the issues involved in clinical research. Content is presented clearly and concisely, using straightforward language. It delineates relevant concepts for students and also serves as a quick reference for practicing nurses.

We believe that for research to be meaningful, a working knowledge of the research process is a prerequisite. Therefore we realize the importance of research vocabulary and are cognizant of the fact that terms such as statistical significance, null hypothesis, random sampling, experimental design, and multivariate analysis many times confuse the research consumer or novice investigator. Therefore, when explaining the research process we give careful attention to the use of charts, tables, and other summary techniques. This serves to highlight major content areas in a utilitarian way. In addition, the book includes suggested readings at the end of each chapter as well as a glossary of commonly used research terminology at the end of the book.

Nurses may find that in addition to being consumers of research, they may also be involved in conducting research or research-like activities. They may want to design a product evaluation, conduct a small pilot study, or compile a staff survey. For this reason *Nursing Research for Nursing Practice* also contains material that may be useful in the design and conduct of small studies. Readers are therefore assisted to meet practical, realistic objectives.

This book is structured into five units. Unit I, Introduction to Research, provides a framework for subsequent chapters. Unit II addresses the planning stages of a project, ranging from the review of literature to the actual design. In Unit III are chapters concerned with implementation, that is, data collection, measurement, and sampling. The evaluation of results is highlighted in Unit IV. Finally, Unit V considers aspects of research that are concerned with practical factors that may facilitate or impede the translation of research into a practice setting.

The major distinguishing feature of this book is its emphasis on the practical clinical application of the research process. A richness of clinical understanding is evident throughout, reflecting our continued commitment and involvement in clinical nursing practice. Research utilization—a topic given only cursory (if any) attention in similar texts—is afforded an entire chapter. Another chapter is devoted to practical realities of research in the clinical arena. The issue of research ethics is more comprehensively covered than in similar texts.

Nursing Research for Nursing Practice is not intended to offer comprehensive coverage of all facets of the research process. This we gladly relinquish to standard reference texts. Instead we wish to assist our readers to meet practical, realistic objectives, namely to be able to appreciate research as a lively, integral part of the professional role.

KARYN HOLM

JANE LLEWELLYN

Acknowledgments

We wish to acknowledge Dr. Luther Christman for teaching us to value research as the cornerstone of clinical practice. We would also like to thank the following persons for reviewing our manuscripts and providing insightful suggestions:

Joan Adams, MSN, Virginia State University, Petersburg, Virginia
Sylvia Britt, MSN, DSN, University of Alabama—Birmingham, Birmingham, Alabama
Diane Elliott, RN, EdD, State University of New York—College at Brockport, Brockport, New York
Anita Fields, PhD, McNeese State University, Lake Charles, Louisiana
Joyce Keithley, RN, DNSc, Rush University, Chicago, Illinois
Evangeline Lane, PhD, Georgia State University, Atlanta, Georgia
Anna K. Leach, PhD, Incarnate Word College, San Antonio, Texas
Patricia A. Martin, RN, BSN, MS, Miami Valley Hospital, Dayton, Ohio

Special appreciation goes to Dr. Anna Leach who compiled the accompanying Instructors Manual.

In addition, Karyn Holm wishes to acknowledge Dr. Marjorie Powers for her mentorship; and her family, Terry Holm and Robert and Kathryn McGaghie, who have always supported her efforts.

Jane Llewellyn would like to acknowledge Dr. Shirley Fondiller for maturing her writing interests; Steve Wozniak for providing the technology; and her family, John and Elizabeth for their love, support, and encouragement, and Margaret Gentry and the late Howard Gentry for instilling the value of knowledge.

Contents

INTRODUCTION TO RESEARCH

This unit contains two chapters. The first chapter, titled "What Is Research?" differentiates research from other types of inquiry. It also discusses the role of research in advancing nursing science and practice. Chapter 2, "Overview and Critique of the Research Process," provides a summary of the criteria upon which critique of research is ordinarily based and directs the reader to elements of critique found in summary tables interspersed throughout the book.

What Is Research?

OBJECTIVES

After completing this chapter the reader will be able to:

1. Differentiate research from other problem-solving methods.
2. Give examples of basic and applied research.
3. Discuss the role of research within the discipline of nursing.
4. Describe the relationship of theory and research.

The clinical practice of nursing is beset with a never-ending stream of problems needing solutions. Many problems can be solved by the individual nurse through logical reasoning, experience, or trial and error, or even by relying on custom, policy and procedure, precedent, or tradition. At times nurses seek solutions to problems by consulting an authority, for example a supervisor, a clinical specialist, or a physician.

While the traditional methods of problem-solving are legitimate and desirable in many situations, they are not without limitations. One section of this chapter will describe some of these problems. In addition, some problems are so important, occur so frequently, or are so intriguing that a more formalized approach to problem-solving may be in order. For these problems, the research process can be used to facilitate resolution.

Within the pages of this chapter, the scientific research method is described and its purposes and relation to a theoretical base for nursing practice are discussed. In the ensuing chapters, more specific research procedures and issues are addressed.

DEFINITION OF RESEARCH

Broadly defined, research is any activity whose purpose is to find a valid answer to a question that has been raised. In other words, it is a method of determining truth or knowing. Several approaches to discovering facts qualify under this definition. The scientific method, problem-solving, and the nursing process are all directed toward this end. In effect, these processes are all related, having overlapping conceptual similarities. Each involves identifying information needed to reach a goal, developing a course of action, implementing the plan, and assessing the results.

Clinical practitioners recognize the overlap between practice and research. Every nurse-patient encounter is a problem-solving process. When a nurse interacts with a patient, the situation is assessed, a problem is identified, nursing interventions are planned, the plan is implemented, and finally the results of the interventions are evaluated. Because each encounter is unique and likely to be highly variable, a cookbook approach is not feasible and an informal investigation must be conducted with each individual case.

Table 1–1. PROBLEMS NOT AMENABLE TO THE SCIENTIFIC RESEARCH PROCESS

Questions reflecting judgments
Ethical questions
Moral questions
Value questions
Questions limited by theoretical development
Questions limited by methodological development

Although the term research is sometimes used in these broad contexts, a more specific designation is considered for the purposes of this text. The more formalized view of research refers to structured and systematic investigations designed to test a hypothesis and draw conclusions, thereby developing or contributing to generalizable knowledge. The outcomes of research may be theories, principles, or statements of relationships. Research is characterized by empiricism; that is, its methods can be verified objectively by another investigator.

WHAT IS *NOT* RESEARCH?

Research questions essentially deal with tangible, observable phenomena. Research requires answers whose truth and meaning can be validated by others. Thus, not every question is researchable or amenable to the research process (Table 1–1).

Questions reflecting judgments, ethics, morals, or values cannot be answered through research. For example, determining if abortion on demand is better than the birth control pill in preventing unwanted pregnancies is not possible. What is meant by "better"? Whose value system is to be used? If the question is operationalized (or defined) so that it becomes factual, then it becomes feasible to explore the question through research inquiry. Thus, one could determine the frequency with which each method is used, or one could identify attitudes related to each practice. These approaches thus become matters of fact and can be empirically explored.

Research is also limited by the state of theoretical development. Researchable questions are more difficult to identify prior to the discovery of the essential underlying framework. For example, research directed toward cure of infectious disease was not possible without the essential assumptions set forth in the germ theory.

The absence of adequate methodology may also limit the researchability of a question. Determining exactly how many stars are in the sky might be theoretically possible. However, because instrumentation is not available to determine the number of stars, the question is not researchable.

DIFFERENTIATING RESEARCH FROM OTHER TYPES OF INQUIRY

As stated at the beginning of this chapter, nurses use many varied methods for obtaining answers to their questions. In this section, some of these methods and the advantages and limitations of each are explored.

Logical Reasoning

Logical reasoning or "common sense" combines experience, intellectual faculties, and formal systems of thought. One thinks through problems by using a process of either induction or deduction to arrive at a conclusion. Difficulties can arise with either approach.

When inductive reasoning is used—that is, developing generalizations from specific observations—the quality of the knowledge derived from such an approach is highly dependent upon whether or not the specific examples used as the basis for generalizations are typical of the problem under study. If a nurse drew conclusions about older persons based solely upon her observations of patients with Alzheimer's disease, the result might be the erroneous belief that senility is an inherent factor in the aging process.

Deductive reasoning—developing specific predictions from general principles—can also lead to erroneous conclusions. Since deductive reasoning is dependent upon previously discovered theories, its validity is linked to the truth of the original generalizations. Cultural stereotypes can be the basis of faulty reasoning; if a nurse bases a clinical approach to a Greek patient on the erroneous belief that all

Mediterraneans are hot-headed and emotive, then serious misjudgments may result.

Additionally, neither of these logical reasoning approaches has a mechanism for evaluation as an inherent characteristic. Thus, there is no built-in check for the truth of the conclusion.

Experience

Most nurses at one time or another have worked with another nurse who had so many years of experience that she was able to solve most routine problems based upon her past encounters with similar situations. This individual invariably knew just the right approach or technique to a successful resolution because she had experienced that particular problem previously and had worked through the solution at that time.

Although it is often said that "there is no teacher like experience," this approach does have its drawbacks. When only experience is relied upon to solve problems, people tend to repeat old ways and it is less likely that one will explore new possibilities. Hence, individuals who rely only upon experience eventually will become stagnant and less adaptable to a rapidly changing environment.

Faulty conclusions can also result from experience if an individual's experience is too restricted to allow her to develop accurate generalizations. Further, knowledge obtained in this manner is haphazard, unsystematic, and unrecorded and thus not ordinarily accessible to others.

Tradition, Custom, Precedent, Habit

Problem resolution using tradition relies on custom, precedent, and habit for the answers to questions. "We've always done it this way" reflects the essence of this approach. The nursing policy and procedure manual often includes some of these elements.

There are several reasons why this approach is so often used. First, tradition is very efficient; each person does not have to begin anew to understand a particular phenomenon. Secondly, it facilitates communication because it provides a common foundation of reference for multiple members of a group.

The drawback to relying on these methods is that they usually have not been evaluated. The fact that patients with myocardial infarctions have been denied ice water over the years does not necessarily mean that ice water is harmful for cardiac patients. How many nursing policy and procedure manuals contain directives that are not based on analyzed data?

An added problem with tradition is that it frequently interferes with the possibility of change and contributes to stagnation of practice rather than encouraging innovation. Research differs from tradition in that research is based on tested reasoning rather than on ritual.

Authority

A common method of finding answers to questions or solutions to problems involves consulting another person who has expertise in a well-defined area. A nurse who has a clinical problem relating to a patient's ileoconduit might call an enterostomal therapist for assistance. The rapid accumulation of knowledge and technological changes within health care have made it impossible for any one practitioner to be expert in all areas. The result is the evolution of the concept of specialists. The advantages in terms of economy of time and in the quality of information are obvious.

The problem with authorities is that they are not infallible. When one relies heavily upon the advice of authorities, one takes the risk that the authority is not always correct. Beyond that, the authority is not always readily available. Another problem is that reliance on authority leads to blind obedience rather than eliciting understanding and questioning.

Trial and Error

Trial and error is akin to informal experimentation. One encounters a problem, tries an intervention, and, if the intervention works, adopts it as a solution. If it isn't effective, an alternate approach is tried until the problem is successfully solved.

The drawback to trial and error as a dominant approach to problem resolution is that it is fallible and further it is inefficient. Much time can be expended attempting to resolve a question that has already been adequately addressed by another practitioner. Research differs from trial and error because it is planned in such a way that it can be replicated by others.

In summary, although we use these problem-solving methods from time to time, they all have the important limitation of restricting knowledge to a narrowed scope. Knowledge gained by these methods is often inaccessible to others who may face the same or similar problems. Thus, these approaches do not contribute to the overall body of nursing science.

Beyond the limitation of narrowed scope, we must be cognizant of the inherent risk we take when we call upon these methods of resolution. Our solutions to problems may not be optimal, and they may even be detrimental and counterproductive. The scientific research method is the best way to assure that questions are addressed objectively and rigorously.

TYPES OF RESEARCH

Basic Research

Basic research is that which is conducted to establish fundamental facts or to develop or test theory. It is sometimes said that basic research is aimed at producing new knowledge, while applied research is undertaken to find solutions to practical problems (Table 1–2). Results from basic research are usually not in a form that is directly applicable to clinical practice.

The Division of Nursing of the Bureau of Health Professions, Health Resources and Services Administration (U.S. Department of Health and Human Services) calls this level of research in nursing "fundamental" research and explains that it is research that addresses or focuses on the biological and/or behavioral functioning of human beings, their environments, and their social systems. It constitutes the scientific base from which nurses or other clinical professionals can develop and test theories. From this fundamental pool of knowledge are drawn the theories upon which clinical intervention strate-

Table 1–2. EXAMPLES OF BASIC AND APPLIED RESEARCH

	Definition	**Example**
Basic research	Establishes fundamental facts or tests theory	Studying the attitudes of teenage mothers toward their babies
Applied research	Tests the use of facts or theories within nursing practice	Testing an intervention designed to increase bonding between teenage mothers and their babies

gies and different practice methods can be based. Some examples of fundamental biological and/or behavioral research that has been funded by the Division of Nursing include studies on the responses of children to pain, the perceptions of the elderly concerning their physical functioning and health care needs, the effects of radiotherapy on cancer patients, and the effects of caffeine on the outcomes of pregnancy.

Applied Research

Within nursing, applied research—or nursing practice research, as it is termed by the Division of Nursing—focuses on nursing interventions, procedures, techniques, and/or methods of patient care. These activities may be technical, physical, verbal, cognitive, psychosocial, and/or interpersonal. Examples of practice research funded by the Division of Nursing have included studies on endotracheal suctioning of critically ill patients, nurses' attention to psychological distress among medical-surgical patients, the effect of nurses' empathy on patients, and the effectiveness of prenatal care provided to Navajo women.

Because nursing is an applied science, we often borrow knowledge from other basic sciences, such as physiology, anthropology, sociology, immunology, and others. Other applied disciplines, such as dentistry, engineering, medicine, and social work have done likewise. More recently, however, nurse researchers have been conducting basic research as well. Both types of research are necessary to the advancement of professional nursing practice.

PURPOSES AND GOALS OF NURSING RESEARCH

The overall purpose of research for any profession is aimed at discovering the truths of the discipline. What is the body of knowledge and how can it be used to the advantage of practitioners? More specifically, research can be conducted to describe phenomena, discover relationships among phenomena, explain phenomena, predict phenomena, and control phenomena. The goal of nursing research is to facilitate the development of clinical nursing interventions that will improve health outcomes and contribute to the optimal delivery of health care. According to the American Nurses' Association, nursing research "develops knowledge about health and the promotion of health over the full life span, care of persons with health problems and disabilities, and nursing actions to enhance the ability of individuals to respond effectively to actual or potential health problems" (American Nurses' Association, 1981). Nursing research complements biomedical research, which is primarily concerned with causes and treatments of disease.

APPROACHES TO REASONING

Just as there is more than one way to skin a cat, there is more than one method to approach problem resolution. Basically, there are two overall ways in which a situation can be explored, induction and deduction. Table 1–3 shows examples of inductive and deductive reasoning approaches.

Induction

An inductive approach, or inductive reasoning, is a process of reasoning that starts with facts about specific situations and attempts to

Table 1–3. EXAMPLES OF INDUCTIVE AND DEDUCTIVE RESEARCH

	Definition	Research Example
Inductive reasoning	Reasoning from the particular case to the more general abstraction	A nurse observes the behavior of hospitalized children and concludes that the childrens' separation from their parents is very stressful
Deductive reasoning	Reasoning from the general abstraction to the particular case	A researcher knows that separation anxiety occurs in hospitalized children and then predicts that the children in hospital X whose parents do not room in will manifest symptoms of anxiety

establish general propositions. It is reasoning from the particular case to a more general abstraction. Inductive research is also sometimes referred to as a phenomenological approach.

For example, a nurse may make specific observations about the behavior of certain mastectomy patients and come to the conclusion that *in general* these women are dealing with changes in body image. Through an inductive approach to theory-building, a researcher observes certain patterns, trends, or associations among phenomena and then uses these observations as a basis for explanation or prediction.

Deduction

A deductive approach, or deductive reasoning, is a process of reasoning that starts with given premises and attempts to derive valid conclusions. It is reasoning from the general abstraction to the particular case.

For example, if we know as a general principle that anxiety inhibits learning, we might deduce that the preoperative patient who is highly anxious concerning surgery will benefit less from the nurse's teaching of proper postoperative behaviors than the patient who is less anxious. We might further deduce that a nursing intervention designed to reduce preoperative anxiety would result in better learning.

THE ROLE OF THEORY IN ADVANCING SCIENCE AND PRACTICE

Definitions of Terms

In order to discuss the relationship between theory and nursing research, it is necessary to identify and define key terms.

Concept. A concept is an abstract idea that represents a class or group of things or actions having certain characteristics in common. Consider for example the concept of pain. When a nurse talks about pain, she is not really communicating an *actual* experience, but a highly simplified and generalized version of it—an interpretation that reflects the professional consensus regarding the essential attributes of "pain." The actual conscious experience of the event is infinitely more specific with regard to intensity, location, duration, quality, and precipitating factors than the message communicated by this generic use of the term "pain." If one actually tried to communicate a detailed cognitive experience, it might take a lengthy explanation but would still not completely express in words many of its more subtle nuances.

Concepts enable us to simplify and organize our environment and to communicate efficiently with others. For example, the physical therapist views ambulation chiefly as a physical act involving specific muscle groups. The nurse is likely to have a different concept of ambulation involving factors related to improving circulation, ventilation, and morale in addition to the physical act of moving about. However, the nurse and the physical therapist normally have enough agreement on the critical attributes of their concept of ambulation to enable them to work together and communicate with each other.

Principle. A principle is a statement of relationship between two or more concepts. A principle is similar to a proposition, postulate, premise, law or axiom. Although all of these terms have slightly different meanings and usages, they all describe the kinds of linkages that exist between concepts.

Hans Selye's description of the stress syndrome can be used to illustrate what is meant by a principle. He believed that a person's body responds to the nonspecific demands of stress by means of the general adaptation syndrome, which continues until adaptation occurs or death ensues. The general adaptation syndrome consists of three phases—the alarm phase, the phase of adaptation or resistance, and the phase of exhaustion. The concepts that form the basis of Selye's description include stress, general adaptation syndrome, general defense mechanisms, and specific defense mechanisms. His description postulates that relationships occur between stress and the body's defense mechanisms, which are activated to cope with the stress.

Theory. A theory, although defined in many different ways, may be thought of as an abstract generalization that presents a systematic explanation about the relationships among phenomena. A theory is a series of principles, or propositions, regarding the interrelationships among concepts. Thus, concepts and principles are components of a theory.

Selye's description of the stress response is a theory. It is composed of several general concepts that are linked by a set of statements or principles, which in turn serve to explain the phenomenon of stress. Theories can be extensive enough to describe and explain large segments of human experience. On the other hand, theories can be restricted in scope, focusing only on a narrow range of phenomena.

Model. A model is a simplified, symbolic (sometimes graphic) representation of a theory or conceptual scheme. Since a word or phrase can convey different meanings to different individuals, a visual or symbolic representation of a theory or conceptual framework often helps to express abstract ideas in a more readily understandable or precise form than the original conceptualization. In essence, a model is an attempt to represent reality with a minimal use of language. As the old phrase goes, "a picture is worth a thousand words."

Purpose of Theory

What purpose does theory serve in the real world? The overall objective of theory is to make scientific findings meaningful and generalizable—to explain why things are the way they are. Scientifically validated facts in isolation from one another remain isolated pieces of data. Connections must be made between these facts in order for their application to life situations to have meaning.

The analogy of a jigsaw puzzle can be used to illustrate the point. Apart from one another, the pieces are meaningless. However, when logically related to each other, the pieces take on new meaning and allow visualization of a total picture that was previously not evident.

Einstein's theory of relativity is a good example. Einstein used pieces of existing knowledge and proposed previously unthought-of relationships between those known scientific facts. The result was his theory, which allows application of that knowledge in revolutionary ways.

The Relationship Between Theory and Research

The relationship between theory and research may be conceptualized as a double helix, similar to DNA (Fig. 1–1). Fawcett (1978, p. 50) states:

> Theory is one helix spiralling from the conception of an idea through modifications and extensions to eventual confirmation or refutation. Research is the second helix, spiralling from identification of research questions through data collection and analysis to interpretation of findings and recommendations for further study. The core of the double helix is the pairing of theory development with the research process. In the core, theory directs research and research findings shape the development of theory. It is this core that avoids the potential triviality of the separate helices.

Theory and research—one is essential for the other. That is, theory can be developed and tested only by using research. Research findings clarify and validate concepts and principles and thus build and test theory. Theory enhances understanding of phenomena through the structure it provides. In research this increased understanding allows us to formulate new research questions and hypotheses and analyze problems using a theoretical perspective. Put another way, results of research serve to develop and validate theory, while theory as it is developing and being validated constantly

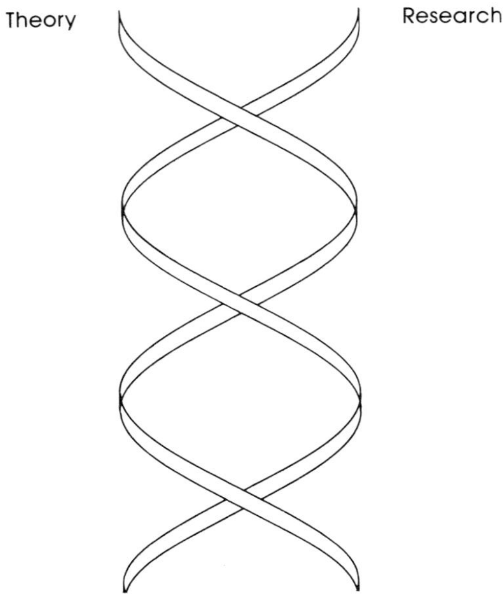

Figure 1–1. The double helix of theory and research.

generates new research questions and provides new perspectives for examining "old" questions.

Can theory and research exist separately? Does all theory need to be tested? Must all research be based upon theory? One need only look at the literature to observe that theory and research are not always linked. Fawcett (1978, pp. 56–57) further states:

> Many failures to integrate theory and research occur when the research impetus is pragmatic and the scientist does not bother to develop a theory to explain results. Such research may be very important in practical terms, but it is likely to be sterile and not advance the discipline. However, a theoretical interest can also get in the way of integration when scientists put all their energies into constructing elegant theoretical edifices which they do not trouble to test, or which, even worse, may be untestable.

Another point should be made concerning the interrelationship of theory and research. A research study rarely tests a grand theory in its entirety. More than likely, one study tests only a small portion of a theory. Thus, it takes many research studies—each building upon the other—to support the overall theory. In effect, each segment of research is likely a piece of a puzzle and each piece may be the key to fitting others into place. Thus, it is important for scientists to take care to relate their studies explicitly to the larger body of knowledge in the discipline. "Only when theory and research are integrated do both become nontrivial; and only then can they contribute to the advancement of science" (Fawcett, 1978, p. 49).

Questions and Activities

1. *Consult a dictionary for a definition of "research." How does this definition (or these definitions) correspond to your conceptualization of nursing research? To the A.N.A. definition of "nursing research"?*
2. *What are the similarities and differences between research and problem-solving?*
3. *Suppose a nurse is interested in trying a new approach to patient teaching. Briefly explain how she might use each of the following methods in arriving at different teaching strategies:*
   a. *Logical reasoning*
   b. *Experience*
   c. *Authority*
   d. *Trial and error*
   e. *Research*
4. *Consult a current issue of a nursing research journal. For each study reported, decide whether you believe it is basic research or applied research. Do your opinions change if you use the definition of "fundamental" research as specified by the Division of Nursing, Department of Health and Human Services?*
5. *Referring to a physiology textbook, read a description of the gate control theory of pain. What is this theory? Can you identify the concepts, principles, and models within this theory?*

Bibliography

American Nurses' Association (1981). *Research priorities for the 1980's: Generating a scientific basis for nursing practice.* (Publication No. D–68). Kansas City, MO: American Nurses' Association.

Ausebel, D. P. (1968). *Educational psychology: A cognitive view.* New York: Holt, Rinehart, and Winston.

Batey, M. V. (1971). Conceptualizing the research process. *Nursing Research, 20*(4), 296–301.
Fawcett, J. (1978). The relationship between theory and research: A double helix. *Advances in Nursing Science, 1*(1), 49–62.
Hardy, M. E. (1978). Perspectives on nursing theory. *Advances in Nursing Science, 1*(1), 37–48.
Jacox. A. (1974). Theory construction in nursing. *Nursing Research, 23*(1), 4–13.
Kaplan, A. (1964). *The conduct of inquiry*. Scranton, PA: Chandler.
Schlotfeldt, R. M. (1975). The need for a conceptual framework. In P. J. Verhonick (editor). *Nursing research*. Boston: Little, Brown.
Stevens, B. J. (1979). *Nursing theory*. Boston: Little, Brown.

2

Overview and Critique of the Research Process

OBJECTIVES

After completing this chapter the reader will be able to:

1. Discuss the process of critiquing research.
2. Specify elements to consider in evaluation of each component of the research report.

As preparation for entry into the nursing profession you must learn what research is all about. As a practicing professional nurse you will be expected to keep abreast of new knowledge both within and outside of nursing by attending conferences and by reading reports of studies in various professional journals. Publication of a research report often carries an aura about it that may lend credibility and an air of respectability to a project that may not necessarily be deserved. That is why it is important for nurses to be discriminating about what studies are worthy of application, and this requires knowledge and skill in research critique.

This book will help you become an intelligent consumer of research. At the end of each chapter are tables listing elements for critique to help you identify strengths and weaknesses of studies and to make comparisons among studies offering similar but conflicting findings. In addition, we have provided a glossary of key research terms to help you in your analysis of research.

Remember, critique is not a negative word. It means to assess strengths and weaknesses and make decisions concerning applicability of findings to clinical practice. One should remember that the goal of critique is not to find flaws and mistakes; certainly weaknesses and limitations may be identified in all studies, especially those conducted in a clinical setting. Rather, the goal of critique is to undertake an objective and thoughtful evaluation of the content of a study and its potential for contribution to clinical practice knowledge.

Stetler and Marram (1976) suggest a model for evaluating research findings for their applicability to clinical practice. The first step involves determining the strength of the research design (validation) through a traditional critiquing process. Secondly, a comparative evaluation of the study must be undertaken to determine what variables affect the decision to change practice and how likely it is that one would be able to implement a study's findings. Finally, once it has been established that a study can feasibly be applied, the nurse is ready to decide whether or not to apply the findings to a particular situation. These essential phases of the model are illustrated in Figure 2–1.

HOW TO PROCEED

Much information about the credibility of a study can be surmised before even reading the first word. First, note the journal in which

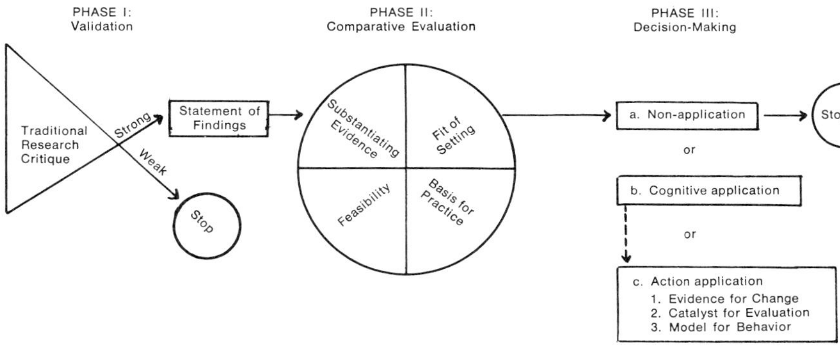

Figure 2–1. A model for the utilization of research findings in nursing practice. (From Stetler, C., and Marram, G. (1976). Nursing Outlook, *24*:559–563.)

the article has been published. Does the publication adhere to high standards? The hallmark of a scholarly journal is a distinguished editorial board that oversees peer review of published articles. As a research consumer you should become familiar with the primary research journals within nursing and your related clinical fields. These are discussed in Chapter 12.

Another point to consider before actually reading the article is the credibility of the author. Does the author have the credentials, consultants, and/or work experiences to be able to conduct an investigation rigorously and knowledgeably? We would not think too highly of a study of surgical techniques if it was conducted by a psychiatrist. Similarly, we should look to the education and clinical expertise of nurse researchers to ascertain their credibility in carrying out a particular study. (However, just as publication of an article does not necessarily mean that it is a great study, neither does a Ph.D. or a D.N.Sc. guarantee that a nurse is a great researcher.)

The timing of a study is another important element. The date of publication is not the date when the study was conducted. Because many journals now have lengthy backlogs before an article is published, they will often indicate on the first page when the article was accepted for publication. Some studies will also indicate the time during which the study was implemented. Critically evaluate this date. Were there significant external factors that may have influenced the findings? For example, a survey of retention factors in nursing employment would need to be viewed in light of the economic

Table 2–1. STEPS IN THE RESEARCH PROCESS

Formulation of the research problem
Review of the literature
Formulation of the conceptual framework
Description of concepts and variables
Formulation of objectives, questions, and/or hypotheses
Description of the design
Description of the population and sample
Development of the methods for data collection
Analysis of data
Interpretation of results
Communication of findings
Recommendations
Conclusions

conditions at the time of data collection. Other types of studies may be less influenced by concurrent events or by the passage of time.

Where does one begin when evaluating a research article? It is important to know how a research report is structured. While every report is unique, emphasizing different aspects of the research process, in general almost all will follow a common roadmap (Table 2–1). This sequence usually begins with a statement and discussion of the research problem and proceeds to a description of the study methods and procedures, then to data analysis and, finally, to discussion of the findings. As a research consumer one is often tempted to read only the results of a study without looking first at the purpose and the methods. Remember a chain is only as strong as its weakest link, and by skipping directly to the conclusions you may miss important factors that influenced the credibility of the results.

Although each reader usually develops personal preferences about how to proceed with reviewing an article, many will follow a particular sequence. A logical place to begin is to read the abstract, if one is included. (As you will learn in Chapter 12, an abstract is a brief summary of the study and its results found at the beginning of an article.) The abstract will give you the highlights of the project. You can then skim the article, paying special attention to figures and tables to get an overall idea of the project. If it seems relevant and of interest, the reader can proceed with a more careful and critical reading of the report in its entirety. Then it is a good idea to reread the abstract to ascertain an accurate understanding of the study. It is important to avoid the temptation to read only the beginning and end of an article. By so doing, a reader may make erroneous assumptions about what ensued in between and may either act on findings that are not based upon sound methods or, equally unfortunate, may disregard an article when in actuality much could have been learned from knowing the methods that were used.

PROBLEM STATEMENT

As you will discover, one of the most important parts of a study is a clear, concise problem statement. It is critical that each study be placed within the framework of previous investigations and that the author demonstrate how the present study will advance knowledge in the area. Findings derived from a study without a clearly defined problem may not be findings you are willing to apply to your practice.

The statement of the research problem will also usually provide the reader with the hypotheses of the study. These should be simply and unambiguously stated so that the reader has a clear idea of the dependent and independent variables and the target population to whom the findings will be generalized.

A review of the literature is another important element of placing the research problem into context. Be sure to note if the cited works are relevant to the study, authoritative, complete, and current.

METHODS

Sound methodology (sampling, design, procedures, data collection instruments) is critical. To make judgments, one must know the process and techniques used to arrive at conclusions. A study with poor methodology accompanied by strong conclusions and recommendations is not one that can advance nursing knowledge. Without a knowledge of methodology one will not know whether to place any faith in the results.

A key element in the methodology is a description of the sampling techniques. A critic will be concerned with the appropriateness of the sample for the hypothesis or question. In addition, it is important that the sample be representative of the population and that the population be specifically defined.

Another important factor in the methodology is the choice of research design. Did the design reflect the research questions, and was it adequate to control the variables?

The choice of data collection instruments and methods will also be crucial to the quality of the study. Were they measuring what they were intended to measure in a way that was consistent? Other important elements to evaluate in relation to the methods include the training of assistants, the conduct of pilot studies, and the degree to which human rights have been protected.

Finally, has there been sufficient description of all of the procedures and methods? A good key to evaluating this is to ask yourself if another researcher would be able to repeat the study under comparable conditions.

RESULTS AND CONCLUSIONS

Evaluation of a study's results begins with assessment of whether or not they are presented in a clear and understandable manner. Are tables and graphs accurate and adequately explained? A good table should be able to stand alone and be clearly understood. Were the statistical tests appropriate to the hypotheses, and were levels of significance stated?

Following the results, the researcher should draw conclusions about the meaning of the data. These conclusions should be logical and follow from the stated purpose of the study. The author should also suggest implications for practice and for further research.

The ultimate evaluative question in a critique is, "Are the findings worth the conduct of the project?" Answering this question involves determining the study's significance to practice and the advancement of knowledge in the field. It may be said that "Any study not worth doing is not worth doing well!" In other words, a study may have been stunningly executed, using the highest of standards and the most sophisticated of techniques, but if it adds nothing to nursing knowledge, it probably should not have been conducted.

Do not be fooled into thinking that because a study cost thousands of dollars and had hundreds of subjects, results should be used without scrutiny. Bigger is not necessarily better. There have been many small studies that were clearly conceived and executed that have produced very credible results. When deciding what studies you will use and which researchers you will believe, it is important that you be aware of the factors that will affect the credibility of a study. This book will give you such necessary information.

ELEMENTS FOR CRITIQUE

Specific elements for critique, which are also listed and discussed within the following chapters in this book, are summarized below.

RESEARCH PROBLEMS AND HYPOTHESES: (Chapter 3)

- Is the problem clearly stated?
- Are key variables identified?
- Does the background logically lead to the problem by demonstrating gaps in knowledge?
- Is the relationship of the present problem to previous research clear?
- Is the problem significant?
- Can the problem be tested?
- Does the introduction to the problem lead from the general to the specific?
- Is it a problem relevant to nursing?
- Does the problem imply possibilities for empirical testing?
- Can the problem be feasibly tested?
- Is the problem appropriately narrow without being trivial?
- Are the hypotheses, research questions, and/or objectives clearly stated?
- Does the researcher clearly state what is not being studied as well as what is?

REVIEW OF LITERATURE: (Chapter 4)

- Were the investigators qualified to conduct the particular type of research?

- Does the conceptual framework suggest relationships among variables?
- Are the important findings of others clearly delineated?
- Were primary sources used?
- Are classic studies cited from authorities in the field?
- Does the bibliography reflect that reasonable sources of related literature have been investigated?
- Is the review logically and clearly organized?
- Has adequate credit been given to the ideas and works of others?
- Is the review limited to the key areas related to the problem under study?

VARIABLES: (Chapter 5)

- What variables are defined in the study?
- Are there any undefined variables?
- Are key variables reflected in the problem statement and/or hypotheses?
- Are all significant variables defined in clear, precise terms?
- Are operational definitions used when appropriate?
- Are independent and dependent variables carefully delineated?
- Have intervening or extraneous variables been considered?

RESEARCH DESIGN: (Chapter 6)

- Is the design clearly indicated?
- Is it appropriate to the problem?
- Is there sufficient knowledge of the problem to warrant the design?
- Does the design control for or minimize the extraneous variables that may affect the results of the study?
- How does the design control for threats to internal or external validity?
- What modifications, if any, could be made in the research design to improve it without significantly increasing the time and money required to carry out the study?
- Will it be possible for other researchers to replicate the research design of the study?

RESEARCH INSTRUMENTS: (Chapter 7)

- Are the data collection instruments clearly described?
- Was adequate rationale given for instrument selection?
- Were the instruments appropriate measures of the variables under study?
- Do the instruments measure data at the appropriate level of measurement?
- Is there evidence of satisfactory validity and reliability?
- Are validity and reliability reassessed for the specific population under study?
- Are the instruments pre-tested?
- Are the instruments consistent with the abilities of the subjects?
- Is there evidence that research personnel were trained in the use of the instruments?
- Is the time required for administration of the instrument realistic?
- Were the instruments administered in the same way to all subjects?
- Are the limitations of the instruments addressed?

MEASUREMENT: (Chapter 8)

- Are key variables quantified?
- Is the level of measurement described?
- Are there data to support the reliability of the measures?
- Are there data to support the validity of the measures?
- Is the level of precision of measurement consistent with the intent of the study?
- Are sources of measurement error acknowledged?

SAMPLING: (Chapter 9)

- Does the researcher clearly describe the sampling procedure?
- Is the sample random or nonrandom?
- Are randomization procedures adequate?
- Does the researcher describe the representativeness of the sample to the population?
- Is the sample size adequate?
- Is there evidence of selection bias?

- If a nonrandom sample is used, is the distribution of key variables assessed?

ANALYSIS OF DATA: (Chapter 10)

- Are descriptive statistics used for all key variables?
- Is there evidence of non-normal distribution? That is, are standard deviations larger than the means?
- Are statistics appropriate to the level of measurement?
- Are statistical values reported?
- Are degrees of freedom reported?
- Are violations of underlying statistical assumptions addressed?
- Do the statistical procedures clarify, enhance, and address the research questions?
- Was the most effective statistic chosen?
- Was the level of significance reported?
- What consideration was given to Type I error?
- Was a bivariate procedure used when a multivariate procedure would have been more appropriate?

INTERPRETATION OF RESULTS: (Chapter 11)

- Are results interpreted in light of the original study problem?
- Do results coincide with expectations?
- Are results linked to previous research?
- Are results grounded in data?
- Are both negative and positive findings reported?
- Are weaknesses in the data honestly addressed?
- Are generalizations appropriate?
- Is practical significance addressed?
- Are conclusions justified?
- Are limitations clearly spelled out?
- What recommendations are made for implementation and further study?

REPORT OF RESULTS: (Chapter 12)

- Does the title of the study reflect key variables?
- Is there a clearly stated, brief abstract?

- Is the report logically organized?
- Is the bibliography related to the central theme?
- Is there clear documentation of others' work?
- Is the format consistent throughout?
- Has the investigator been honest in reporting results?
- Is the study reported in sufficient detail to allow replication?
- Is the report written in a professional style?
- Is non-sexist language used?
- Are tables, graphs, and charts used to enhance text?
- Is the report written in an interesting manner?

PROTECTION OF HUMAN RIGHTS: (Chapter 14)

- Has the risk-benefit ratio been considered?
- Are the procedures ethical?
- Is informed consent obtained?
- Are provisions made to protect populations at risk?
- Are privacy and anonymity safeguarded?
- Are subjects free to withdraw from the study at any time?
- Is there evidence that the study was approved by appropriate review boards?
- Are efforts made to minimize risks to subjects?
- Is there evidence that the researcher has made provisions for needed care and treatment when appropriate?

SUMMARY

The process of research critique involves a judgment of the strengths and weaknesses of the research problem, the methodology, and the results and conclusions. It is important to remember that critique is both a science and an art. This chapter briefly reviews the scientific criteria upon which research critique is ordinarily based. The art of critique, however, is equally important. It involves the critic being sensitive to the individual researcher, keeping in mind that the criticism is directed at the product and not at the person.

Questions and Activities

1. *Select a current nursing research report. Critique it according to the guidelines suggested in this chapter.*
2. *See if you can locate a study from another discipline similar to the one examined in number one above. How does the critique of this study compare?*
3. *How can research critique be a part of peer review?*
4. *Discuss the differences between critiquing a written research report from a journal and critiquing an oral report of research.*
5. *Suppose that you have presented a study at a research seminar. Role-play with a classmate an interchange of criticism concerning the report. Remember that critique focuses on both positive points and areas for improvement.*

Bibliography

Davitz, J. R., and Davitz, L. L. (1977). *Evaluating research proposals in the behavioral sciences.* 2nd edition. New York: Teachers College Press.

Fleming, J. W., and Hayter, J. (1974). Reading research reports critically. *Nursing Outlook, 22*(3), 172–175.

Haughey, B. P. (1984). Considerations in applying research findings to practice. *Dimensions of Critical Care Nursing, 3*, 288–292.

Jacox, A., and Prescott, P. (1978). Determining a study's relevance for clinical practice. *American Journal of Nursing, 78*(11), 1882–1889.

Leininger, M. (1968). The research critique: Nature, function and art. *Nursing Research, 17*(5), 444–449.

Schantz, D., and Lindeman, C. A. (1982). Reading a research article. *Journal of Nursing Administration, 12*, 30–33.

Stetler, C., and Marram, G. (1976). Evaluating research findings for applicability in practice. *Nursing Outlook, 24*, 559–563.

PLANNING A RESEARCH STUDY

Unit II is concerned with planning a study. The initial focus is on defining a specific research problem. Next, the review of the literature places the research problem into context. Then the different types of variables are discussed with emphasis on control of extraneous variables using design and statistical measures. This unit concludes with descriptions and examples of various designs utilized in nursing research.

3

Research Problems and Hypotheses

OBJECTIVES

After completing this chapter the reader will be able to:

1. Describe sources of research problems.
2. Differentiate between research hypotheses and questions.
3. Discuss the essential criteria for research problems.

Defining a research problem is not as easy as it may appear. Expressing an idea in researchable terms is a critical prerequisite to planning and implementing any research project. This chapter will discuss the factors associated with formulating a researchable problem.

EVOLVING RESEARCH INTERESTS

Where do research problems originate? One of the most important aspects of identifying a research problem is the interest the researcher has in the topic. Research is a lengthy process, and for someone without true interest in a topic it can become quite a tedious endeavor. There is no hard and fast rule pertaining to how one can insure that research problems are interesting. One can only hope that interest is sustained from the inception of the idea to the writing and presenting of the final report.

Identifying research problems is enhanced by becoming increasingly familiar with a topic. Therefore an initial step is to use the library to determine what has been written in both books and journals and to immerse oneself in the topic. Then one might increase understanding of the topic by communicating the information to others. This may be done in one of the following ways.

Volunteer to Conduct an Inservice Program. Presenting the topic in an informal way to a small group is an ideal approach. When an inservice program is conducted in a conference room, the group is usually small and discussion is a natural consequence. Such discussion can clarify and modify ideas about the research topic. Furthermore, to prepare an inservice presentation requires that thoughts and ideas be organized.

Write an Article for Publication. Writing a paper forces one to outline main ideas and thus helps in identifying where more information is needed. Gaps in knowledge may be your own or may represent real voids in what is known by others in the scientific community. This can help delineate a research direction. If the paper is accepted for publication, another benefit is derived. Those who read the article will link your name to the topic, thus enhancing your credibility.

Use Creative Approaches to Problem Identification. Creativity, as you may be aware, involves using a thought process that takes one outside of one's "modus operandi," that is, outside of usual patterns and routines. Going beyond our hospital units or offices and exposing ourselves to new people with differing ideas not only helps to broaden our exposure but also helps us to think in new ways.

Increase Your Contact with Those Outside of Nursing. Those outside of nursing can help to shed new light on old ideas. For example, learning what those in medicine or pharmacology think about treating decubitus ulcers may lead you to designing a study testing a new nursing protocol.

Become Professionally Involved. Become an active member of professional organizations. At meetings you will meet others from outside your hospital or college and have an opportunity to exchange ideas. Professional contacts are invaluable, and you may find someone who has similar research interests.

Participate in Workshops, Conferences, and Conventions. Attending workshops, conferences, and conventions, both intra- and interdisciplinary, serves to broaden your horizons and your ability to think creatively. There is also a need to attend some professional gatherings outside one's own geographic area to increase the chances of exposure to different regional ways of doing things.

Read Professional Journals. Being a regular reader of journals helps one to see what others think is important and the areas in which there is research activity. Here one is given the opportunity to be exposed to the thoughts and ideas of those who live in other parts of the country or even the world.

Read Novels and Other Books. Your leisure-time reading may have a significant bearing on how you think about the world. Professional writers are creative thinkers and can teach us a great deal about what it means to move beyond the here and now and extend our imagination. Robert Ludlum and Irving Wallace are examples of contemporary authors who have taken what they have imagined and transformed it into a reality for readers.

GENERATING RESEARCH HYPOTHESES, QUESTIONS, OR OBJECTIVES

Outlining the Problem

Research hypotheses, questions, or objectives evolve from a clear and concise problem statement. The beginning of a research report should introduce the problem in a general way and evolve to a specific statement of the problem. A problem is supported by the literature, which should demonstrate gaps in knowledge and place the problem within this context.

The characteristics of a strong research problem are similar to those of a strong legal defense. The defense begins by placing the problem within the framework of contemporary knowledge. It is introduced in a general way and then gaps in existing knowledge are discussed. Then concessions are given; that is, points that really are not in favor of the researcher's position are acknowledged. Note here that a strong problem is characterized by few concessions. From concessions the problem evolves to points in favor of the researcher's position, in other words, the defense of the problem.

If you are not the researcher but are the research consumer, check to see if the researcher has followed such guidelines, which are the hallmarks of a strong research problem. Remember that a strong problem is the most essential part of any research report. When you are to be the researcher, it would serve you well to outline your statement of the problem so it flows from the general to the specific; from gaps in existing knowledge; and from points not in favor of your position to those points in your favor.

How the Specific Problem is Stated

Once the general problem area is presented and arguments are delineated, a specific problem statement is needed.

In the declarative (or positive) form a problem is stated as a purpose. Table 3–1 cites specific examples of problem statements in the declarative form. In the interrogative form problems are stated as a question (Table 3–2). In the declarative form the specific problem statement begins with "the purpose of this study is. . . ." When the interrogative form is used, the problem is posed as a question.

Because problem statements guiding the majority of studies should identify specific variables, definitions of the variables are needed. Table 3–3 gives an example of a specific problem statement and corresponding definitions of variables. Note that a variable can be a characteristic, phenomenon, concept, or thing that has the capacity to vary. We will be learning more about specific kinds of

Table 3–1. SPECIFIC PROBLEM STATEMENTS (DECLARATIVE FORM)

Research Focus	Problem Statement
Knowledge of medical terminology among hospital patients	To determine if there continues to be a difference between the staff's perception of patients' knowledge of medical terminology and the actual knowledge of patients in a health care setting. (Byrne and Edeani, 1984)
Morale and perceived control in the elderly	To identify patterns of causal relationships among perception of situational control, socioeconomic status, health, functional dependency, length of institutionalization and morale. (Ryden, 1984)
Influence of coronary artery bypass surgery on quality of life	To assess how coronary artery bypass surgery influences subjective and objective aspects of quality of life early in the recovery period following bypass surgery. (Penckofer and Holm, 1984)

Table 3–2. SPECIFIC PROBLEM STATEMENTS (INTERROGATIVE FORM)

Research Focus	Problem Statement
Stress and coping in neonatal intensive care nurses	What are the major classes of coping strategies reported by neonatal nurses? Are reported coping strategies influenced by the relative stressfulness of the events? Are reported coping strategies influenced by the nurse's characteristics of age, basic educational preparation, and clinical experience? (Jacobson, 1983)
New graduate adaptation	Will there be a difference in the adaptation of new graduates who use educational modules during hospital orientation and new graduates who do not? (Weiss, 1984)
Arthritic patients and causal thinking	To what extent will arthritics construct causes for their condition? (Lowery, Jacobsen, and Murphy, 1983)

Table 3–3. DEFINITIONS OF VARIABLES

Study Problem	Definitions of Variables
What is the effect of therapeutic touch without physical contact on state of anxiety of hospitalized cardiovascular patients? (Quinn, 1983)	*Therapeutic touch* was defined as using the hands to direct excess body energies from a person playing the role of healer to another person for purposes of helping or healing. *State of anxiety* was defined as a transitory emotional state or condition of the human organism characterized by subjective, consciously perceived feelings of tension, apprehension, and heightened autonomic nervous system activity.

variables in Chapter 5. Without clear definitions of variables it is virtually impossible to decide if the results of one study can be easily compared with those of other studies.

Criteria for Research Problems

When a problem is important to nursing, the findings will generate further study and help build nursing knowledge. The American Nurses' Association Commission on Nursing Research (1982) has identified research priorities for the 1980's. The priorities shown in Table 3–4 have been generated to assist the profession in developing knowledge to improve practice and advance the profession. Research priorities have also been identified by other professional groups such as the American Association of Critical Care Nurses (Lewandowski and Kositsky, 1983), the Oncology Nursing Society (Oberst, 1978), and the New York State Nurses Association (Oberst and colleagues, 1981).

Although a problem may be very important, practical constraints may preclude it from being researchable. The study, no matter how important, will be impossible to conduct if subjects, equipment, or facilities are unavailable; if there is little cooperation from key people, as for example physicians who will discourage patients from participating; if the researcher has little experience; or if there are insufficient funds to carry out the project.

Examples of Problem Statements

The following examples from the nursing research literature are intended to illustrate how researchers have arrived at specific problem statements. Each begins with a general overview of the problem area, presents a defense of the study problem, and ends with a specific problem statement.

Dressler, Smejkal, and Ruffolo (1983) compared oral and rectal temperatures in patients receiving oxygen by mask. To introduce the topic, reference is made to the importance of vital signs in assessment.

Table 3–4. RESEARCH PRIORITIES IDENTIFIED BY THE ANA COMMISSION ON RESEARCH

Practice
Studies to reduce complications of hospitalization and surgery (sleep deprivation, anorexia, diarrhea, neurosensory disturbances, respiratory infections, circulatory problems, and others).
Studies to improve the outlook for high-risk parents and high-risk infants.
Studies to improve the health care of the elderly.
Studies of life-threatening situations, anxiety, pain, and stress.
Studies of adaptation to chronic illness and the development of self-care systems and group care systems.
Studies to facilitate the successful utilization of new technological developments in patient care.
Studies of nursing interventions to promote health.
Studies to facilitate the successful application of new knowledge to patient care.
Studies to define and delineate healthy states.
Studies of addictive and adherence behaviors.
Studies of under- and overnutrition.
Studies to evaluate the outcomes and/or effectiveness to consumers and providers of different patterns of delivery of nursing services.
Profession
Studies of manpower for nursing education, practice, and research.
Studies of quality assurance for nursing and studies of measures of criteria for practice and education.
Studies of the cost effectiveness of nurse utilization and preparation in relation to: acute care, long-term care, and community health.
Studies in the history and philosophy of nursing.
Studies of nursing curriculum.
Studies of the organization of the nursing profession.

Body temperature in the postoperative cardiac surgical patient is then addressed, and the common practice of employing rectal temperatures in these patients is then cited. The researchers then argue that taking rectal temperatures precipitates increases in incisional pain and general discomfort but that nurses assume that rectal temperatures are more accurate. In an attempt to disprove or validate this assumption, the study was conducted to determine whether a difference exists between oral and rectal temperatures in cardiovascular surgical patients receiving oxygen by mask.

When studying trends in development and behavioral styles in low birth weight infants, Medoff-Cooper and Schraeder (1982) introduce the problem by stating that low birth weight infants are a challenge to nurses practicing in both inpatient and outpatient settings. They go on to say that follow-up data on low birth weight infants are sparse and not easily used by the clinician. In the review of the literature they point out that the results of previous studies are inconsistent. Therefore, the purpose was to investigate the developmental characteristics of the very low birth weight infant and subsequently to explore the behavior of the preterm infant and its impact on the parent-child relationship. Their specific research questions were designed to seek a relationship between specific variables, as for example the relationships between very low birth weight and infant development, and between very low birth weight and infant temperament.

RESEARCH HYPOTHESES

There are two types of hypotheses, research hypotheses and null or statistical hypotheses. Research hypotheses focus on specific aspects of the research problem and are used to test existing theory. They are written in present or future tense, include only one relationship or difference to be tested, and allude to the population of interest. In a study of consensus about the marital relationship during transition to parenthood, Broom (1984) stated five hypotheses, all of which appear in Table 3–5. All are written in the future tense and suggest empirical testing. Each includes only one difference and identifies a specific population, namely spouses. Null or statistical hypotheses are hypotheses claiming no significant difference or relationship. Research hypotheses should not be confused with null hypotheses. Please note, however, that every research hypothesis has a corresponding null hypothesis, which is never proved directly. A null

Table 3–5. RESEARCH HYPOTHESES

I. Prenatal predictions of the most important postpartum concerns will differ from those actually identified as most important in the postpartum period.

II. Husbands and wives will disagree on the relative importance of postpartum concerns, both prenatally and postpartally.

III. Husbands and wives will perceive greater agreement between themselves regarding the relative importance of concerns than actually exists.

IV. Postpartum couples will be more accurate in estimating their spouses' rankings than prenatal couples.

V. Couples will communicate relatively more about concerns they consider most important.

From Broom, B. L. (1984). *Nursing Research* 33(4), 223–228.

ELEMENTS FOR CRITIQUE OF RESEARCH PROBLEMS AND HYPOTHESES

- Is the problem clearly stated?
- Are key variables identified?
- Does the background logically lead to the problem by demonstrating gaps in knowledge?
- Is the relationship of the present problem to previous research clear?
- Is the problem significant?
- Can the problem be tested?
- Does the introduction to the problem lead from the general to the specific?
- Is it a problem relevant to nursing?
- Does the problem imply possibilities for empirical testing?
- Can the problem feasibly be tested?
- Is the problem appropriately narrow without being trivial?
- Are the hypotheses, research questions, and/or objectives clearly stated?
- Does the researcher clearly state what is not being studied as well as what is?

hypothesis is either rejected or not rejected to support or not support a research hypothesis. We will be learning more about null hypotheses in our discussion of statistical tests.

While research hypotheses are always part of an experimental study, they are not absolutely necessary for other kinds of studies. Many times researchers not planning an experiment will choose to focus their research problem by generating research questions or stating research objectives.

Questions and Activities

1. *Compare the Lewandowski and Kositsky priorities for research in critical care nursing with Oberst's priorities in cancer nursing research. How do these compare with priorities established by the ANA Commission on Research?*
2. *Differentiate between hypothesis and research question. Discuss whether one is more important than the other.*
3. *Identify at least five researchable nursing problems relevant to your area of clinical interest.*
4. *State how the above problems might be formulated into hypotheses.*
5. *Select a current research report using hypothesis testing. Determine the extent to which the hypothesis was supported or not supported. Could the study have been conducted without using hypothesis testing?*

Bibliography

Broom, B. L. (1984). Census about the marital relationship during transition to parenthood. *Nursing Research, 33*(4), 223–228.

Byrne, T.J., and Edeani, D. (1984). Knowledge of medical terminology among hospital patients. *Nursing Research, 33*(3), 178–181.

Commission on Nursing Research (1980). Generating a scientific basis for nursing practice: Research priorities for the 1980's. *Nursing Research, 29*, 219.

Dressler, D.K., Smejkal, C., and Ruffolo, M.L. (1983). A comparison of oral and rectal temperature measurement on patients receiving oxygen by mask. *Nursing Research, 32*(6), 373–375.

Fuller, E.O. (1982). Selecting a clinical nursing problem for research. *Image, 14*(2), 60–61.

Jacobson, S.F. (1983). Stresses and coping strategies of neonatal intensive care unit nurses. *Research in Nursing and Health, 6*(1), 33–40.
Lewandowski, L.A., and Kositsky, A.M. (1983). Research priorities for critical care nursing: A study by the American Association of Critical-Care Nurses. *Heart and Lung, 12*(1), 35–44.
Lowery, B.J., Jacobsen, B.S., and Murphy, B.B. (1983). An exploratory investigation of causal thinking of arthritics. *Nursing Research, 32*(3), 157–162.
Medoff-Cooper, B., and Schraeder, B.D. (1982). Developmental trends and behavioral styles in very low birth weight infants. *Nursing Research, 31*(2), 68–72.
Neuman, M.A. (1982). What differentiates clinical research? *Image, 14*(3), 86–88.
Oberst, M.T. (1978). Priorities in cancer nursing research. *Cancer Nursing, 1*, 281–290.
Oberst, M.T., Ventura, M., Fredrickson, K., Schmidtt, M., Noel, N., Corless, I. (1981). Nursing research priorities identified by the New York State Nurses Association. *Journal of the New York State Nurses Association, 12*(1), 21–25.
Penckofer, S.H. and Holm, K. (1984). Early appraisal of coronary revascularization on quality of life. *Nursing Research, 33*(2), 60–63.
Quinn, J.F. (1983). Therapeutic touch as energy exchange: Testing the theory. *Advances in Nursing Science, 6*(2), 42–49.
Ryden, M.B. (1984). Morale and perceived control in institutionalized elderly. *Nursing Research, 33*(3), 130–136.
Weiss, S.J. (1984). The effect of transition modules on new graduate adaptation. *Research in Nursing and Health, 7*(1), 51–59.

4

Review of Literature

OBJECTIVES

After completing this chapter the reader will be able to:

1. Describe the purposes of the literature review.
2. Cite categories of supporting references.
3. Discuss steps in the literature review process.
4. Relate how the written literature review is organized.

The literature search and review is a crucial portion of the research process. It frequently means the difference between a targeted, thorough, and well-designed study and one that is fragmented, diffuse, and loosely planned. A good literature review, though sometimes difficult and painful to produce, can ultimately save valuable time and can spare the researcher costly and/or embarrassing mistakes.

For many investigators, the literature search is the most enjoyable and most challenging portion of a study. In this phase, one is free to explore an idea, to investigate it from multiple perspectives and to tease out the various elements for investigation. It can be a time when an investigator has the self-indulgent luxury of exploring the library and delving deeply into a subject of interest.

PURPOSES OF THE LITERATURE REVIEW

Conducting a literature review serves several functions. These are summarized in Table 4–1 and described in the following paragraphs.

Source for Research Ideas. Sometimes one reviews the literature to obtain ideas for problems to investigate. A nurse on a cardiac unit may have an interest in a particular area of patient care, such as teaching of patients. She may know that she wants to design an investigation to look at an aspect of patient teaching but may not have the idea narrowed any further. By reading studies in the general area, she may develop ideas for new hypotheses or find that the studies reviewed actually contain proposed hypotheses for further research. Studies that produce surprising or unexpected findings can frequently generate further questions.

Orientation to What Is Known. When an idea for a study is formulated, it is necessary to determine what aspects of the particular problem have already been investigated. Very few ideas are entirely original. More than likely, the exact problem or a very closely related

Table 4–1. PURPOSES OF THE LITERATURE REVIEW

Source for research ideas	Defining the variables
Orientation to what is known	Guiding the design and methods
Defining a conceptual context	

area has already been studied. Even when little has been formally explored in an area, it is necessary to establish a baseline of what is known to date about the problem. A researcher does not want to make the mistake of overlooking key investigations in the field.

Defining a Conceptual Context. It is important for all scientific investigation to fit within an identified theoretical or conceptual scheme. The value of a conceptual model as a guide to research is described in Chapter 1. By surveying the literature, the investigator can identify relevant theories and models that have potential utility for the study being proposed.

Defining the Variables. The literature can be helpful in delimiting and refining the variables relevant to a problem. A researcher may wonder if sex or age, for instance, make a difference in a particular treatment approach. By looking at previous studies, she may be able to determine that sex has not been demonstrated to make a difference, but age has been a strong predictive factor. She can then design the study to control for these variables more appropriately than she could have without that information.

Guiding the Design and Methods. A researcher can save time and headaches by going to the literature before designing the methodology of a study. It is possible to identify instruments already available, developed and tested by others, that could be used. In addition, problems and pitfalls that have been encountered by other researchers can be uncovered and potentially avoided. The literature survey can also highlight information about the potential sample, its characteristics, and how likely it will be to obtain the proposed sample. Methods of data analysis that have been used in previous studies are also evident in a literature survey.

Sometimes help with methodology can come from unexpected sources. A literature search should not be confined to the subject area of the study being proposed. By expanding the search to areas that use similar methodologies, areas that address similar variables, or areas that investigate similar populations, one can often obtain valuable suggestions and can identify approaches that need only minor modifications to be adaptable to one's own study. For example, an investigator interested in studying muscle tension in childbirth may find helpful information in studies of migraine headaches, because the electromyographic technique would be very similar for both studies.

CATEGORIES OF SUPPORTING REFERENCES

References are not all the same. Some are more helpful than others because of their inherent validity or the strength of their evidence. In the following section, the various types of data sources are reviewed (Table 4–2).

Anecdotal Reports. Professional journals are replete with articles that describe clinical phenomena. They can take the form of case studies, clinical impressions, observations of situations, or descriptions of programs. Generally, these sources of information are limited to one or two situations or patients. They most often are naturally occurring events, so they do not generally reflect control of variables as do more formally designed studies. While there is strong value to case studies and single-subject research designs (as we shall see in Chapter 6), these approaches generally do not weigh as convincingly as evidence as do larger, more controlled studies.

Anecdotal reports do serve a very useful purpose, especially in relation to generating hypotheses and suggesting variables for study. In addition, it is important to encourage publication of anecdotal reports because they are more timely; an important finding can be brought to public awareness much more quickly than it could via a larger formalized study. It is perfectly acceptable to include anecdotal reports in a literature review, so long as they are balanced with evidence of a stronger nature.

Theories and Models. As discussed in Chapter 1, theories and models can be used as supporting references. A theory, model, or conceptual framework may guide the researcher in identifying or defining the variables of a study, or the model may suggest hypotheses.

Primary Data Sources. Primary data sources are those in which the data are reported by the person or group that actually gathered the

Table 4–2. CATEGORIES OF SUPPORTING REFERENCES

Anecdotal reports
Theories and models
Primary data sources
Research studies
Statistical reports
Secondary data sources

information. There are two broad types of primary data sources, research studies and statistical reports. Research studies range in scope from the small pilot study to broad-based, controlled experiments. A familiar example of a statistical report is census data. From information collected by the Census Bureau, one can obtain demographic information about a block, a standard metropolitan statistical area (SMSA), a county, a state, or the nation as a whole. Other examples of primary statistical reports include reports about disease prevalence from sources such as the Centers for Disease Control, the World Health Organization, the National Cancer Institute, or the National Heart, Lung and Blood Institute.

Secondary Data Sources. Secondary data sources are those in which the reporter of the information is not the person or group that actually obtained the data. A common example of a secondary data source is the published literature review. In a published review, a person knowledgeable in the field compiles, reviews, summarizes, and analyzes a grouping of publications in a related field. The published review can be extremely helpful to the novice researcher, especially in providing an overview and in guiding the researcher to classic works.

Secondary reports are another typically encountered example of a secondary data source. Novice researchers must be very careful to avoid assuming that an official-sounding report is a primary data source. The Surgeon General's reports, for example, are typically a compilation of published evidence on a specified problem. The data are not actually obtained by the Surgeon General. Another example of a secondary report can be reports from non-profit health organizations such as the American Heart Association. These also are typically compilations of data collected by others that address a particular area of concern.

It is permissible to use secondary works in a literature review. However, as with anecdotal reports, they should not be the sole sources and should be balanced with primary sources. The researcher must always remember that the use of secondary sources carries a big risk: one must trust that the reviewer has presented a thorough and unbiased review of the facts, a task not easily accomplished even with the best of intentions. Each person or group is likely to have a vested interest, a hidden agenda, or a personal bias. Unless great care is taken to preserve objectivity, this influence on the review will inevitably become apparent.

Sometimes original works are not available, especially in relation to unpublished theses and dissertations and foreign works. However, a researcher should make every reasonable effort to obtain original works when feasible.

STEPS IN THE LITERATURE REVIEW PROCESS

Conducting a literature review need not be a formidable task if a logical, organized approach is taken. The following steps, summarized in Table 4–3, can serve as a guide for the process.

Become Familiar with the Library. This may seem like an obvious assumption but it bears emphasis. An experienced researcher knows the library and the reference librarian and uses them appropriately. A few key questions to a librarian may sometimes reveal specialized services available that can potentially save hours of tedious work. In addition to services available, it is also important to know about the method of cataloging. Although most libraries continue to have a traditional card catalog, some are now using computer-generated catalog books, microfilm catalogs, or on-line computer cataloging. One also needs to know how books are arranged. Is the cataloging in the Library of Congress system, the Library of Medicine system (Table 4–4), or some other system?

Narrow the Topic. The more delineated a topic, the more useful a literature search is likely to be. Unless a survey is being conducted for the specific purpose of delineating a topic, it is recommended that the topic be suitably self-contained from the beginning.

Check for Appropriate Terminology. It is unlikely that all papers on a given topic will be listed in one place. Therefore, to avoid over-

Table 4–3. STEPS IN THE LITERATURE REVIEW PROCESS

1. Become familiar with the library
2. Narrow the topic
3. Check for appropriate terminology
4. Identify major entry points
5. Group article citations by journal title
6. Scan bibliographies for overlooked titles
7. Retrieve, review, summarize, and critique

Table 4–4. NATIONAL LIBRARY OF MEDICINE CLASSIFICATION SYSTEM

W	Medical profession	WR	Dermatology
WA	Public health	WS	Pediatrics
WB	Practice of medicine	WT	Geriatrics; Chronic disease
WC	Infectious diseases	WU	Dentistry; Oral surgery
WD	Deficiency diseases	WV	Otorhinolaryngology
WE	Musculoskeletal system	WW	Ophthalmology
WF	Respiratory system	WX	Hospitals
WG	Cardiovascular system	WY	Nursing
WQ	Obstetrics	WZ	History of medicine

looking some key works, it is important for a researcher to determine all of the various connections that a topic might have. It becomes necessary for the investigator to play with the subject, taking it apart and viewing it from all sides. In some fields, a thesaurus is available that lists commonly used descriptors. Although there is not a specific thesaurus for nursing, a terminology guide may be found at the beginning of most indexes to nursing literature.

It is helpful to make a list of all of the terms used to describe the subject of interest and keep it handy at all times so that it can be modified as the search progresses. In going through the literature, the researcher is likely to find new descriptors and will also probably discover that some of the original ones are not useful.

Identify Major Entry Points (Table 4–5). One of the hardest and most overwhelming tasks for the beginning researcher in searching the literature is knowing where to start. Coming face-to-face with the thousands of volumes in a library can be formidable if there is no roadmap to lead the search. Following is a description of the entry points most commonly used in guiding a search of the literature.

Card Catalog. Figure 4–1 illustrates an example of a Library of Congress catalog card. Card catalog entries are commonly arranged

Table 4–5. MAJOR ENTRY POINTS FOR A LITERATURE SEARCH

Card catalog	Prepared literature searches
Indexes	Bibliographies
Abstracts	Annual reviews of research
Computer	Review articles

③ ① **NURSING SERVICE, HOSPITAL**
WY
31
Al3e ②Abdellah, Faye G
1958 ④ Effect of nurse staffing on satisfactions with nursing care; a study of how omissions in nursing services, as perceived by patients and personnel, are influenced by the number of nursing hours available, by Faye G. Abdellah and Eugene Levine. Chicago, American Hospital Association ⑤ [1958]
⑥ 82 p. diagrs., tables. 23 cm. (Hospital monograph series, no. 4)
American Hospital Association. Pub[lication] no. G112-58 [i. e. G113-58]
⑦ Report of a study by the Public Health Serivce's Division of Nursing Resources.
⑧ Bibliography: p. 44–46.
⑨ 1. Hospitals—U. S.—Stat. 2. Nurses and nursing—U. S.—Stat. I. Levine, Eugene, joint author. II. U. S. Public Health Service. Division of Nursing Resources. (Series: American Hospital Association. Hospital monograph series, no. 4)
⑩ RA972.A3 362.11⑪ 59—17229
⑫ Library of Congress

Figure 4–1. Example of a Library of Congress catalog card. The circled numbers have been added to indicate the various types of information the card contains, as follows: (1) The subject matter of the book. (2) Author's name. (3) The call number (National Library of Medicine System). (4) The title and subtitle of the book. (5) The copyright date. (6) The number of pages in the book. This book also contains diagrams and tables. (7) A description of the contents of the book. (8) An indication that the book has a three-page bibliography. (9) Categories under which the book will be cataloged. (10) Library of Congress call number. (11) Dewey Decimal call number. (12) Indicates the "publisher" of the card.

by subject, by author, and by title. Many large libraries now have their card catalogs computerized.

Indexes. Not all catalogs and indexes are arranged in the same way. They will all begin with a section that directly or indirectly tells "How to Use This Book." To save time and avoid frustration, it is smart to begin by reading this section. Some examples of indexes are listed in Table 4–6.

Abstracts. Examples of commonly used abstracts relevant to health research are listed in Table 4–7. There are two types of abstracts. The most reliable first-hand information is that obtained from abstracts written by the person who originally authored the publication. An example is *Dissertation Abstracts International*, a compilation of abstracts written by the dissertation authors themselves.

A second type of abstract comes from abstracting services that summarize research that has been reported elsewhere. These services

Table 4–6. EXAMPLES OF INDEXES OF NURSING AND RELATED LITERATURE

Cumulative Index to Nursing and Allied Health Literature	International Nursing Index
Current Literature on Aging	Index Medicus
Hospital Literature Index	Science Citation Index
	Social Science Citation Index

are usually set up as a service to professionals in areas where there is such an abundance of research that it becomes difficult for any one person to keep abreast of new knowledge. These sources can be helpful but should be regarded with some skepticism, since they are secondary data sources. They should be used only to guide an investigator to original work.

Computer. Computer-assisted searches, though sometimes involving nominal expense, can be extremely worthwhile, both in saving time and in assuring the completeness of a search. Many computerized bibliographic databases are now accessible. Table 4–8 lists a representative sampling of databases relevant to nursing studies.

A search can be directed by topic area within a specified set of sources of information and within a specified time period. A computer search is not helpful in initial explorations. It is best used when a problem is rather well-defined, so a preliminary manual search is advised.

In computer searches the key terms, or descriptors, are pivotal to

Table 4–7. EXAMPLES OF ABSTRACTS RELEVANT TO NURSING AND RELATED HEALTH TOPICS

Abstracts of Health Care Management
Behavioral Medicine Abstracts
Child Development Abstracts and Bibliography
Dissertation Abstracts International
Excerpta Medica
Feeding, Weight and Obesity Abstracts
Hospital Abstracts
Nutrition Abstracts and Reviews
Pastoral Care and Counseling Abstracts
Psychological Abstracts
Social Work Research and Abstracts
Sociological Abstracts

Table 4–8. COMPUTERIZED BIBLIOGRAPHIC DATABASES RELEVANT TO NURSING STUDIES

*AGELINE: Citations to literature on aging.

*AMA/NET SOCIO/ECONOMIC BIBLIOGRAPHIC INFORMATION: Citations to articles on the non-clinical aspects of health care, including economics, education, ethics, international relations, legislation, political science, psychology, public health, medical practices, and sociology.

BIOETHICSLINE: Citations to the literature on abortion, euthanasia, human experimentation, recombinant DNA research, and numerous other moral, ethical, and policy issues.

*BIRD: Citations to the worldwide literature on the health of children and families. Covers nutrition, sanitation, health education, emotional health, and social factors relating to child and family health, particularly in developing countries.

*CANCEREXPRESS (EXPRESS): Citations to selected journal articles on cancer.

*CANCERLIT: Citations to the worldwide literature on oncological epidemiology, pathology, treatment, and research.

*CANCERNET (INTERNATIONAL DATABASE ON ONCOLOGY): Citations to literature on oncology.

CINAHL (NURSING & ALLIED HEALTH LITERATURE INDEX): Citations to articles in nursing and allied health disciplines. Corresponds to *Cumulative Index to Nursing and Allied Health Literature.*

*DRUGINFO and ALCOHOL USE/ABUSE: Citations to materials that deal with the educational, sociological, medical, and psychological aspects of alcohol and drug use/abuse.

*EMBASE (formerly EXCERPTA MEDICA): Citations to the worldwide biomedical literature on human medicine and areas of biological sciences related to human medicine.

*EMCANCER: Citations to the worldwide literature on cancer.

*EMHEALTH: Citations to the worldwide literature on public health.

*EPILEPSYLINE: Citations to the worldwide literature on all aspects of epilepsy.

HDOK: Citations to reports on aids for disabled persons. Primary coverage is for speech impairment, visual impairment, incontinence, motor disorders, and mental retardation.

HEALTH PLANNING AND ADMINISTRATION: Citations to topics relevant to the provision of health care services, including budgeting, finance, organization, administration, management, planning facilities, and personnel resource development.

MEDLINE: Citations to the worldwide biomedical literature, including re-

Table continued on opposite page

Table 4–8. COMPUTERIZED BIBLIOGRAPHIC DATABASES RELEVANT TO NURSING STUDIES *Continued*

search, clinical practice, administration, policy issues, and health care services.

*NIMH (NATIONAL INSTITUTE OF MENTAL HEALTH): Citations to the mental health literature.

*OCCUPATIONAL SAFETY AND HEALTH (NIOSH): Citations to literature on occupational safety and health. Covers hazardous substances, toxicology, and workplace safety.

*POPLINE: Citations to the worldwide literature on family planning and population. Includes research in human fertility, contraceptive methods, and others.

SOCIAL SCIENCES INDEX: Citations to articles and book reviews in periodicals in the social sciences. Includes anthropology, economics, sociology, psychology, and political science.

*Includes abstracts of citations.
Data from *Directory of online databases* (1984). 5(3), Santa Monica, CA: Cuadra Associates.

the success of the search. An experienced reference librarian can be a helpful ally at this point. A descriptor that is too broad will yield a needlessly large list of references, whereas one that is too narrow may overlook key sources. For example, suppose a nurse is interested in studying the role of patient teaching in decreasing patients' postoperative stress levels. Simply requesting articles on "stress" or even on "patient teaching" will produce a listing that is far more comprehensive than needed. However, when the word "and" is included the search is narrowed to the articles of interest, "patient teaching and stress." With this logic, one might conclude that it would be useful to narrow the search even further to "patient teaching and stress in the surgical patient." This is not necessary and would be too restrictive, since it is likely that articles dealing with patient teaching and stress with any group of patients would yield helpful information. Generally, using three or more simultaneous descriptors severely narrows a computer search.

Literature Searches. Prepared computerized literature searches on topics considered to be of wide interest are available from the National Library of Medicine at no charge (Sparks, 1984).

Bibliographies. Bibliographies are generally more comprehensive in scope and coverage than literature searches since they are usually a result of a combination of manual and computerized searching. Bibliographies are often more extensively annotated. The National Library of Medicine also has an extensive bibliography series (Sparks, 1984).

Annual Reviews of Research. Many professions develop mechanisms to review critically, on a regular basis, the work that leads the discipline forward. These reviews are generally compiled annually in books and are excellent starting points for identifying relevant research. Although nurse researchers should not limit themselves to nursing literature, the *Annual Review of Nursing Research* (Werley and Fitzpatrick) is a recommended starting point. (An example of the contents of initial volumes of this review may be found in Appendix B).

Review Articles. A lucky break is to find a recent survey or review article on the topic of interest. This can be most helpful in providing orientation and key references. However, it should never be used as the sole source of references.

Group Article Citations by Journal Title and Note Bibliographic Information. The format for citations depends upon the purpose of the research. If the research is for an academic requirement, a thesis or dissertation, for example, the university probably specifies a style manual. If the report is being prepared for a particular journal or publisher, there is a specific style guide recommended in most cases. If one is selecting one's own style manual, the related field may be a matter to consider. For example, if a nursing research study seems likely to be of particular interest to clinical psychologists, then the *Publication Manual of the American Psychological Association* might be appropriate.

Scan Bibliographies for Overlooked Titles. Read reference lists of articles and book chapters that deal with the proposed topic. Frequently retrograde searches lead the researcher to earlier material and little-known works.

Retrieving, Reviewing, Summarizing, and Critiquing. It may seem obvious, but it is necessary to write down what one finds in a literature survey. If one is not disciplined to the habit of always writing down the author, title, and page number of each reference, the price may be paid at a later date when endless hours need to be spent tracking down an obscure reference.

Each note or summary should include the following information in some form (Table 4–9):

1. The problem: State the problem and describe any context or setting that makes this problem unique.
2. The design: Use standard terms. Indicate the type, method, and size of the sample, and the population or reference to which findings will be generalized. Include the presence or absence of controls.
3. Data collection methods: Describe instruments, validity, reliability, and interrater training. Include how, when, and where data were collected.
4. Data analysis: Describe how data are organized and statistical techniques used.
5. Findings and/or conclusions: Delineate the results of the study.
6. Recommendations: Include recommendations for further study, for improving research techniques, and for changes in clinical practice.
7. Brief critique: Address whether the researcher's conclusions were justified, whether the findings can be integrated into a theory, and whether there were specific defects or flaws in the design.

The format of notes is a matter of personal preference. The debate over whether to use index cards or notebooks is not as crucial as deciding on a personally useful system and sticking to it. Notebooks offer the advantage of being more compact and easier to transport. On the other hand, cards afford more flexibility when it comes time to arrange the information into a written summary. A compromise approach is putting note materials into bound card "books" (looseleaf binding) now commonly available. These offer the flexibility of having individual cards and also the security of having all the materials bound together.

Table 4–9. KEY POINTS TO BE INCLUDED IN A LITERATURE SEARCH NOTE

The problem under study	Recommendations of the author
The design of the study	Brief critique
Data collection methods	Bibliographic information
Data analysis	Coding indication
Findings and/or conclusions	

Whatever the form of the notes, it is essential to adopt some system for creating order as you go so that you will be able to sort, select, and make sense of the information at some later point. This involves using a coding system that serves as a rough key or index to the information you have obtained.

It is essential to have some system whereby materials can be organized. A collection of notes soon becomes unmanageable; unless a system is adapted from the beginning, retrieval of the information at a later point will be difficult if not impossible.

Several coding systems are possible. One might use a topical system (e.g., coronary artery disease, etiology, detection, treatment, rehabilitation). Another approach is a functional classification (e.g., attitude scales, designs, sampling techniques). Most people probably prefer a combination of the two.

The coding and sorting of information can be a science unto itself. For very large projects there are systems whereby punched cards and machine sorters can be applied.

One standard rule applies: *Whatever the note format or the coding system, write on only one side of the page.* If both sides of a page are used, the process of sorting and arranging the materials is not possible. In the same vein, it is helpful to limit cards or notes to a single thought, topic, or idea. Multiple topics on the same card present similar problems in sorting and arranging.

It is not advisable to take lengthy verbatim notes from the various data sources. However, should some verbatim quotes be used, it is necessary to develop a system for indicating their sources.

Verbatim notes result in several undesirable outcomes. First, it is basically a clerical function; one might as well use a photocopier. If lots of verbatim notes are taken, it is merely postponing the thought and synthesis that must occur at some point. Beyond that, however, when copying exact passages, a researcher does not necessarily need to think about what is being written. On the other hand, if the researcher paraphrases points as they are retrieved, several things happen. The thought is more likely to become ingrained and remembered because an active process has occurred. Plagiarism is less likely to occur because the researcher consciously puts thoughts into his own terms, and a beginning of a first draft for the written report is begun.

Experienced researchers find that note-taking combined with photocopying can be very effective. Within copyright restrictions, you may want to copy a study's abstract and tape it to the back of the notecard. You may also choose to photocopy specific figures or detailed charts or tables rather than write them out by hand. Remember, however, that piles of photocopies of complete articles merely postpone the work of summarizing and synthesizing.

Once a system is adopted, it should be held to consistently. Any system works best when it becomes an ingrained habit.

ORGANIZING THE WRITTEN LITERATURE REVIEW

Beginning researchers often mistakenly think that they need to document and recount everything that has been written or studied in relation to a particular topic. Others are of the notion that the literature review is to "prove" that the researcher thoroughly knows the topic. No wonder the thought of writing a literature review can be overwhelming and immobilizing for some! Basically, the written review, whether it be for a project proposal, an academic thesis, or a published research article, should address two major objectives: it should (1) describe the problem and (2) give historical review of the problem.

Each study cited should be briefly summarized. This summary should include brief information about the problem, the design, data collection, data analysis, and findings and/or conclusions. Point out any areas that are unique or not consistent with previous work. Don't stop here. Make a judgment about the value of this work, pointing out strengths and any weaknesses or lack of controls or errors in logic. Summarize how this study fits with your own.

The review of the literature should end with a good summary of all articles reviewed. The summary should include an analysis of any inconsistencies found in the literature and a summary of the evidence to support the rationale for the proposed investigation.

Since organization of the written review can sometimes be overwhelming, particularly if there is a large amount of material to be surveyed, many researchers find it helpful to prepare a summary chart as the first step. An example is shown in Table 4–10. This chart will serve two purposes: (1) it will help the author organize the way the studies fit together, and (2) it will be useful when the study is completed and the researcher wants to see how the present study fits in the overall picture of research in the field.

Table 4–10. EXAMPLE OF A TABLE TO SUMMARIZE STUDIES IN PREPARATION FOR ORGANIZING A LITERATURE REVIEW*

Citation and Clinical Affiliation†	Sample	What Was Measured	Results	Conclusions

*The organization of the chart can be modified to reflect the aims of a specific study. For example, if statistical treatment of data is a critical factor, then a column for data analysis might be needed.

†It is a good idea to note clinical affiliations of studies. In this way, the investigator has a better idea of institutions and geographical regions that are active in the particular area of investigation. Also, it may highlight limitations if all work originates from one team of investigators.

QUESTIONS THAT OFTEN ARISE CONCERNING THE LITERATURE REVIEW

Following are several commonly asked questions relating to literature searches.

1. How much should be included in a literature review? If a literature review continues forever, it no longer serves a useful purpose. Wise selection, rather than all-inclusive coverage, is the preference.
2. What is the difference between a reference list and a bibliography? A reference list includes only those books and articles that were actually cited in the preparation of the article. A bibliography, on the other hand, is a more comprehensive listing of works relating to the background of the problem or works that are recommended reading on the subject. Most journals require reference lists, not bibliographies.
3. How far back should I go? Continue to search as long as you are

finding articles that are of sufficient use or interest. The only other articles that should be included prior to this point are the seminal (beginning) works and classic studies. (You will recognize the latter because they are cited in the majority of subsequent studies.)

4. What do you do when you can't locate a key book? In this modern age, no researcher needs to feel constricted by the confines or limitations of a particular library. If a title is known, most libraries are able to borrow materials from other institutions through inter-library loan. Within limits, microfilming and photocopying can bring almost any reference within reach of even the most isolated researcher.

ELEMENTS FOR CRITIQUE OF LITERATURE REVIEWS

- Were the investigators qualified to conduct the particular type of research?
- Does the conceptual framework suggest relationships among variables?
- Are the important findings of others clearly delineated?
- Were primary sources used?
- Are classic studies cited from authorities in the field?
- Does the bibliography reflect that reasonable sources of related literature have been investigated?
- Is the review logically and clearly organized?
- Has adequate credit been given to the ideas and works of others?
- Is the review limited to the key areas related to the problem under study?

Questions and Activities

1. *Suppose you want to study the problem of confusion in the elderly. What steps would you take to locate current information on this topic?*

2. *What abstracts and indices might contain citations relevant to Diagnostic Related Groups (DRG's)?*
3. *Discuss the difference between a reference list and a bibliography.*
4. *How would you organize a literature review for a study of health promotion in the school-age child?*
5. *Under what circumstances is it permissible to use secondary sources?*

Bibliography

American Psychological Association. (1983). *Publication manual of the American Psychological Association* 3rd edition. Washington, D.C.: American Psychological Association.

Barzun, J., and Graff, H. F. (1977). *The modern researcher* 3rd edition. New York: Harcourt Brace Jovanovich.

Binger, J. L., and Jensen, L. M. (1980). *Lippincott's guide to nursing literature.* Philadelphia: J.B. Lippincott.

Sparks, S. M. (1984). The National Library of Medicine's bibliographic databases: Tools for nursing research. Image, *16*(1), 24–27.

Taylor, S. D. (1974). How to search the literature. *American Journal of Nursing, 74*(8), 1457–1459.

Werley, H. H., and Fitzpatrick, J. J. (1983). *Annual Review of Nursing Research.* New York: Springer.

Westmeyer, P. (1981). *A guide for use in planning and conducting research projects.* Springfield, IL: Charles C Thomas.

5

Variables

OBJECTIVES

After completing this chapter the reader will be able to:

1. Define specific types of variables.
2. Discuss methods for controlling unwanted variables.
3. Relate the importance of operationally defining variables.

Variables are termed such because they have the capacity to vary. This means that more than a single number or value can be used to describe them. A variable takes many forms and might be a trait, an object or item, a characteristic, or just about anything. Variables are studied in isolation or in combination with each other. They can be examined in their natural environment as managerial stress or manipulated to determine if they precipitate a desired effect as a specific nursing intervention. An investigator is not always aware of all of the variables involved in a particular situation. Thus, there are times when unidentified or unwanted variables influence the data that are collected. This chapter will discuss ways variables are used and will provide definitions and examples to aid in designing or interpreting research.

TYPES OF VARIABLES

Independent, Dependent, and Intervening Variables

To understand independent, dependent, and intervening variables requires a time perspective. Independent variables precede and possibly affect dependent variables. For example, a nurse's culture, age, sex, and basic nursing preparation may affect perceptions of a patient's physical pain or psychological distress. In this instance perceptions of either physical pain or psychological distress are the dependent variables, while culture, age, sex, and nursing preparation are the independent variables.

Dependent variables, sometimes called criterion variables, follow and are influenced by independent variables. They will vary in accordance with variations in independent variables. Independent variables can be viewed as the cause and dependent variables as the effect. In an experiment, changes in a dependent variable are measured following manipulation of an independent variable. Consider for example a situation in which the influence of preoperative instruction (independent variable) is evaluated in terms of postoperative days (dependent variable). Here the investigator is seeking to determine if patient teaching in the preoperative period leads to the desired outcome, specifically a reduction in postoperative days.

Figure 5–1. Intervening variables.

Time 1	Intervening Variable	Time 2
Independent Variable	Intervening Variable	Dependent Variable

The dependent variable should reflect the phenomenon being studied and be sensitive enough to detect experimental effects. For example, if investigators were interested in studying the bone loss that comes as a consequence of a week of bedrest, x-rays may not be sensitive enough to detect such short-term changes.

As shown in Figure 5–1, there may be other variables that come between an independent and a dependent variable. Such factors, known as intervening, extraneous, or confounding variables, may or may not influence the relationship between independent and dependent variables. Suppose that researchers were interested in studying the influence of a particular kind of exercise on developing lower extremity muscles. The impact of the independent variable (the exercise) on the dependent variable (muscle circumference) might be influenced by age, sex, weight, or other activities. When intervening variables are present the relationship between variable one (independent) and variable two (dependent) may be increased, remain the same, be lessened, or disappear entirely.

Discrete, Rank Order, and Continuous Variables

In addition to viewing variables within a time framework, variables can also be viewed in terms of their measurement properties. Variables composed of separate and distinct categories are known as discrete variables. Much of the sociodemographic information collected in nursing studies takes a discrete form. Race, sex, education, and occupation can all be categorized as shown in Table 5–1. For each variable subjects will fit into only one category. Note that sex contains only two subsets and thus is also termed dichotomous. Discrete variables are examples of nominal measurement. Nominal measurement is discussed in Chapter 8.

Variables can also be evaluated by rank order, as happens when rank is assigned in measurement. Many psychometric tests rank order

Table 5–1. CATEGORICAL (DISCRETE) VARIABLES

Race	Educational level
Caucasian	Elementary school
Black	High school
Oriental	College
Hispanic	Graduate school
Others	Occupation
Sex	White collar
Male	Blue collar
Female	Professional

variables, as for example a personality test that deems one individual more or less introverted than another.

Weight, height, blood pressure, and temperature are examples of continuous variables. A variable treated as continuous is one in which there are an infinite number of points between each value.

Attribute and Active Variables

There are times when variables are called attribute variables or active variables (see Table 5–2). An active variable is manipulated. An attribute variable is measured. Thus, any variable to which something is done is an active variable and any that is merely observed is an attribute variable. Some variables may never be active variables because they are, by their very nature, attributes. Examples of such variables include personality characteristics, sex, educational level, and intelligence. Some of these attributes cannot be manipulated at all; others, such as educational level, may be subject to changes, but such changes are outside the scope of nursing research, as subjects present themselves for study with these characteristics already in place.

Table 5–2. ATTRIBUTE AND ACTIVE VARIABLES

Active variable:	This kind of variable can be manipulated. Examples include teaching approach(es); dressing technique(s); resuscitation protocol.
Attribute variable:	This kind of variable cannot be manipulated. Examples include age, sex, level of intelligence.

CONTROLLING UNWANTED VARIABLES

Whenever designing or analyzing research employing independent and dependent variables, we must not fail to consider the potential influence of intervening variables. It is an understatement to say that the potential influences of intervening or extraneous variables should be identified and controlled if one truly expects to answer a research question. For example, the variables of age, sex, weight, or activity discussed earlier should be controlled so the effects of the exercise might be isolated.

A study by Shukla (1981) is a good example of how an investigator controlled extraneous variables taking the form of unequal nursing competencies. When studying primary nursing on two hospital units, the potential for bias due to unequal competencies was ameliorated by 6 months of continuing education sessions that included the nursing care process, communications, patient care planning, and assessment and evaluation of patients' physical, social, and psychological needs. In addition to these general sessions, primary nurses were given sessions on primary nursing, the role of primary nurses, and other related topics.

Randomization

Intervening or extraneous variables can be controlled by randomization. Subjects can be randomly selected from an identified population or randomly assigned to a control or experimental group. Thus, error or bias due to unwanted influences is "equally likely" in any of the groupings of subjects. Theoretically, randomization is the best way to control unwanted variables. Both identified and unidentified sources of error can be assumed to be equally distributed. When randomization procedures are used, we expect that in the long run subjects will be equivalent in terms of all variables. In the short run, randomization assumes that each individual or each group has an equally likely chance of introducing undesirable influences. Randomization and associated procedures are discussed in Chapter 9.

If for some reason randomization is not possible, as for example in a clinic with a limited number of patients, or if an investigator chooses not to randomize, extraneous variables can be controlled within the design of a study in one of the following ways.

Selecting a Homogeneous Sample

The extraneous variable can become part of the sample criteria. For example, if age is a factor in the process of wound healing, then it might be wise to place an age restriction on the sample, choosing only those from a specific age group.

Matching Subjects

Matching subjects in terms of critical variables is another common practice. In this instance two subjects are chosen that are like one another in regard to the variable(s) in question. One of the subjects is assigned to the experimental group and the other to the control group to ensure that the groups are equivalent. Although matching may seem a relatively easy way to control variables, it may be difficult to find matching subjects.

Using Design or Statistical Control

Other options for the control of intervening or extraneous variables are afforded by design or statistical control. In the first instance the critical variables are incorporated into the study design as independent variables. This is sometimes referred to as blocking. If the variables of sex and surgical procedure were to be incorporated into a study, the consequence would be a design similar to that shown in Table 5–3. This design blocks on sex and procedure, which have become separate categories. Thus, when results are analyzed there can be an independent assessment of each category.

Similar to blocking is using each subject as his or her own control. This is done by recording baseline measurement of the dependent variable(s) for each subject and taking subsequent measurements at specified intervals. The subsequent measurements are then compared with the baseline measurements for each subject. The baseline measurement is the control. This approach is useful when the issue is how each individual varies across time, rather than how they vary initially.

A purely statistical approach can also be used. Analysis of covariance is the name of the procedure affording statistical control. When this procedure is used, adjustments are made in the post-test measurement of a dependent variable for pre-treatment or pre-intervention differences. We shall be learning more about this procedure later.

OPERATIONALLY DEFINING VARIABLES

Variables are operationally defined when there is a statement as to the activities or instruments an investigator will use to measure them. For example, if blood pressure is an essential variable in a particular study, an operational definition of blood pressure is needed. It must be clear what kind of pressure the investigator is concerned with. It may be venous pressure, mean arterial pressure, or systolic pressure. We must first define blood pressure in conceptual terms. For example, blood pressure may be defined conceptually as the pressure of blood as it flows through an artery. The operational definition then follows and is directed toward delineating how blood pressure will be measured. For example, the researcher might use readings on a sphygmomanometer at the first and fifth Korotkoff sounds according to Heart Association recommendations.

Table 5–3. EXAMPLE OF A DESIGN USED TO CONTROL VARIABLES OF SEX AND SURGICAL PROCEDURE

	Procedure	Pre-Test	Post-Test
Male	Valve Replacement		
	Cholecystectomy		
Female	Valve Replacement		
	Cholecystectomy		

Table 5–4. DEFINING STRESS

	Conceptual	Operational
Physiological emphasis	Stress is the body's response to physical demand	Measured by blood pressure and urinary catecholamines
Psychological emphasis	Stress is a perceived threat to integrity	Measured by an anxiety scale

While this definition gives limited meaning to blood pressure, it gives the meaning intended for purposes of this particular study. The definition is purposely limited and specific. It becomes clear to others how blood pressure was conceptualized and measured so they can not only critique but replicate the study if so desired.

The importance of a conceptual definition preceding an operational definition deserves further emphasis. Stress is a variable that can be defined conceptually from more than one perspective. Because of this, it is very important that a researcher makes clear the exact conceptual emphasis. As shown in Table 5–4, stress defined from a physiological perspective is operationalized quite differently than stress defined from a psychological perspective.

Operational definitions are prerequisite to the study of variables. Scientific investigators must sooner or later face the necessity of

ELEMENTS FOR CRITIQUE OF VARIABLES

- What variables are defined in the study?
- Are there any undefined variables?
- Are key variables reflected in the problem statement and/or hypotheses?
- Are all significant variables defined in clear, precise terms?
- Are operational definitions used when appropriate?
- Are independent and dependent variables carefully delineated?
- Have intervening or extraneous variables been considered?

measuring the variables they are studying. Operational definitions allow researchers to measure variables as they provide instructions on what and how to observe.

Questions and Activities

1. *Differentiate between independent and dependent variables. Describe how a variable such as "stress" might be used as an independent variable in one study and as a dependent variable in another.*
2. *How might extraneous variables bias research results?*
3. *Consider the variable of systolic blood pressure. How could this be used as a rank order, a continous, or a discrete variable?*
4. *Discuss the pro's and con's of the various approaches to the control of variables.*
5. *An operational definition incorporates the approach taken to measurement. With this in mind, discuss how the variable "post-operative pain" might be operationally defined from the following perspectives:*
   a. *Physiological*
   b. *Cultural*
   c. *Psychological*
   d. *Behavioral*
6. *For each of the above perspectives, also give a conceptual definition of pain.*

Bibliography

Kerlinger, F. N. (1973). *Foundations of behavioral research.* New York: Holt, Rinehart, and Winston.

Shukla, R. K. (1981). Structure vs people in primary nursing: an inquiry. *Nursing Research, 30*(4), 236–241.

5

Research Design

OBJECTIVES

After completing this chapter the reader will be able to:

1. Differentiate between exploratory, correlational, and experimental designs.
2. Differentiate between correlation and causality.
3. Discuss historical research.
4. Describe the use of survey research.
5. Identify the role of grounded theory in nursing research.
6. List the threats to internal validity.
7. Enumerate the threats to external validity.

8. Give examples of specific experimental and quasi-experimental designs.
9. Discuss the issues involved in single-subject research.
10. Identify factors involved in selecting a research design.

Research design structures research activities, providing a blueprint for an investigation. The choice of design depends upon the purposes of the study. Generally research is approached from a descriptive or experimental perspective, both of which include specific designs and/or approaches. Studies not experimental in design are called descriptive designs and include exploratory, correlational, and other approaches to research in which a variable is not manipulated. This chapter will begin by discussing descriptive designs and approaches and continue with a discussion of commonly used experimental designs.

DESCRIPTIVE DESIGNS AND APPROACHES

Exploratory Design

When an investigator has little or no knowledge about specified variables, an exploratory approach is taken. If, for example, the intent is to study how children react being separated from a hospitalized parent and little information is available, the research question would seek to determine the variables involved in children's reactions to being separated from a hospitalized parent. An exploratory design is best carried out with observational methods and open-ended questionnaires and interviews. Only when specific variables have been identified is a correlational approach taken.

Correlational Design

Studies examining relationships are correlational in design. The objective is to identify the relationships between at least two variables.

An example of a correlational design is given by Duxbury and colleagues (1984), who quantified relationships of head nurse leadership style with self-reported staff nurse burnout and job satisfaction in neonatal intensive care units. They used three instruments—the Minnesota Satisfaction Questionnaire, the Tedium Scale, and the Leadership Opinion Questionnaire—which were completed by registered nurses employed in neonatal units.

Correlational research is prerequisite to experimental research. Experimental models of other disciplines have been used in nursing without first clarifying how key variables are related. Because correlation precedes experimentation, correlational studies are very important. As a matter of fact, the "state of the art" of nursing research indicates the need for more investigations that are correlational in design.

The Nature of Correlation. Credit is given to Francis Galton (1822–1911) for development of the correlational method. Galton was not interested in supporting specific hypotheses but was intent upon identifying relationships among variables in heredity. He used methods of statistical correlation before the mathematical foundations of correlation were derived by Karl Pearson. As will be explained in Chapter 10, the most common correlational statistic is known as the Pearson product-moment correlation.

Correlational designs aim to specify the relationships between variables. The magnitude of correlation can be any value from -1.00 to $+1.00$. A positive correlation is not any better than a negative one. A positive correlation simply means that as the numerical values on one measurement increase, so do the values on another measurement, as for example the positive correlation between shoe size and height. A negative correlation is a bit different. When two measurements are negatively correlated, when the numerical values obtained on one measurement increase, the numerical values on the other decrease. Two variables that may be negatively correlated are hours without sleep and mental alertness.

Correlation and Causation. Many researchers mistakenly design correlational studies to identify cause and effect relationships between variables. This is incorrect, as *correlation does not prove causality*. For example, if a high correlation is found between the number of uncomplicated deliveries and the employment of nurse midwives in the state of Illinois, one is not in a position to say that the increased use of nurse midwives caused the number of uncomplicated deliveries to increase. While causality may seemingly be supported, a mere correlation does not speak to which variable preceded (caused) the other. One is free to argue from either position or from a position of no causal relationship. Thus, one should avoid inferring causation from a correlation. Not only is information not given concerning which variable preceded the other, but variables can be highly correlated without being causally related. For example, the number of live births in the state of California may be highly correlated to the temperate climate. It cannot be said however, that the temperate climate causes live births.

The value of correlational designs is that they can lead to the discovery of relationships that can then be studied within the context of an experimental design. Before designing an experiment, however, one should give close attention to the degree of a relationship, selecting only those variables that seemingly have the most influence upon the behavior or phenomenon to be studied. This means that if 15 variables are found to be related to breast self-examination, only those with the highest correlations should be selected for experimental manipulation.

Historical Research

Many nursing studies are concerned with reconstructing the past to reach conclusions about events or people. Data are collected from primary and secondary sources. A primary source is one in which the author was a direct observer of the recorded event, whereas a secondary source is one in which the author is reporting the observations of others. A primary source is preferred because it is firsthand evidence. Donahue (1983) used primary sources, such as original documents, articles, letters, and books written by Isabel Maitland Stewart, to document the essential principles of Stewart's philosophy of nursing. All data sources supported the conclusion that Stewart was progressive and utilitarian in her ethical views.

The historical approach is rigorous. After data have been collected, questions are asked concerning the authenticity (external criticism) and the accuracy and relevance (internal criticism) of the data. When the research is conducted properly, appropriate data are collected, verified, and synthesized to place the historical evidence within the context of the past, the present, and the future.

Survey Research

When a study is defined as a survey, the primary purpose is to gather information about a large number of people by collecting data from a few. The word survey comes from two Latin words. *Sur-* is a derivative of the latin "*super*," which means "above" or "beyond." The second portion of the word, *-vey*, is from the Latin "*videre*," which means "to see." Therefore the word survey, directly translated, means to see above or beyond.

A survey design can serve many functions but most often is descriptive either in a correlational or exploratory sense. It must be noted, however, that the design of a survey is very much dependent upon the specific research objectives.

Regardless of specific objectives, a survey should meet certain standards or indicators of quality. One of these is related to sampling. Because a survey aims to describe a population based on information from a select few, it is essential that the sample obtained be representative of the population. Therefore, it is very important that the sample be random in order that generalizations made to an entire population be accurate.

A national mail survey was conducted by Kirchhoff (1982) to describe the current practice of restrictions imposed on myocardial infarction patients. Two mailings were done. The first was directed to the head nurses of the coronary care units and the second to the head nurse and two randomly selected nurses from each unit agreeing to participate. Follow-ups by either telephone or mail yielded response rates of approximately 87 percent for each mailing.

The quality of a survey is also judged by the reliability of the data. Persons who are studied must be depended upon to be truthful. Any suspicion of this not occurring must be acknowledged.

Surveys are flexible and permit a wide variety of data collection techniques. A telephone interview, a face-to-face interview, and a mailed questionnaire are but a few examples. These will be further described in Chapter 7. In addition, surveys can gather information from individuals at a relatively low cost to the researcher, particularly when a mailed survey is used. Caution is warranted, however. The researcher has little control over individual responses to surveys and may be faced with a low response rate. People many times do not return a mailed questionnaire or do not have the time to be interviewed either via telephone or in person. Another issue is that a survey is usually not able to obtain in-depth information about personal opinions, beliefs, or attitudes, particularly when closed response questionnaires are used.

Grounded Theory Approach

Grounded theory is a combination of inductive and deductive methods. It differs from other designs or approaches in important ways. First, a conceptual framework is generated from the data. Second, data collection is often modified according to the evolving conceptual framework, as for example the use of more probing questions if necessary. Finally, rather than following the usual steps in the research process—that is, stating the problem, outlining the method, and collecting and analyzing data—an investigator using grounded theory codes and categorizes pieces of data as they are collected. Then a tentative conceptual framework is generated which is open to modification. A grounded theory research report will present the conceptual framework generated from collected data. Other literature is then used to explain and support the proposed framework.

To investigate how a stepfather is integrated into an existing family system composed of mother and child, Stern (1978) used a grounded theory approach. This was appropriate as the phenomenon had not been previously examined and there was not an existing theoretical framework.

EXPERIMENTAL DESIGN

True experimental designs are characterized by randomization, manipulation, and control. To qualify as an experiment, a study must be designed to employ randomization procedures, manipulation of an independent variable or variables, and control of extraneous variables.

Experimental design attempts to uphold internal and external validity, which will be described in the following sections. Please note that the adequacy of an experimental design is evaluated in light of each of these factors.

Internal Validity

The extent to which alternative explanations of findings can be eliminated is the evidence needed to support internal validity (Table 6–1). The question to be answered here is, did the experimental treatments make a difference? Extraneous variables, if not controlled, may be difficult to separate from the effects of an independent variable. Cook and Campbell (1979) have defined 13 threats to internal validity.

History. Something other than the independent variable may occur between a pre-test and post-test that may bias results. Note that history is used here in reference to events occurring during the experiment. If a knowledge post-test given to cardiac patients following exposure to patient education materials demonstrates an increase in knowledge, it is entirely possible that the experimental variable (i.e., the patient education material) produced the change. However, if at the time of the experiment a television program was scheduled that discussed cardiac risk factors, it would be difficult to know if the knowledge increases could be solely attributed to the patient educational materials. Attempts therefore should be made to keep the intervening history between pre and post measures as similar as possible for all subjects.

Table 6–1. THREATS TO INTERNAL VALIDITY

History	Interactions with selection
Maturation	Diffusion of treatment
Testing	Compensatory equalization of treatments
Instrumentation	Compensatory rivalry
Statistical regression	Demoralization effects
Selection	Local history
Mortality	

Maturation. Subjects themselves can change during an experiment. The kind and degree of change is somewhat dependent upon the length of time between the pre and post measures. Subjects can become fatigued, bored, older, or hungrier. Such possibilities must be considered prior to the implementation of a study and efforts made to avoid such contamination.

Testing. In pre-test, post-test designs the results of the post-test may be influenced by the premeasure, particularly when it takes the form of an examination that is repeated. While this bias cannot be totally erased, efforts must be made to test all subjects in a consistent way within a comparable time frame, and to expect a gain of a few points when a test is readministered.

Instrumentation. When instruments such as electrocardiographic recording equipment, overbed scales and sphygmomanometers are used, their precision and accuracy may change between measurements. Therefore, calibration procedures should be used prior to each measurement period to eliminate this threat.

Statistical Regression. This phenomenon is frequently described in the educational literature and refers to what happens to extreme test scores, either very high or very low, when a test is readministered. Those who initially score very high will tend to score lower at the second testing period. The reverse also occurs. Those who initially score very low will score higher upon retesting. Scores will therefore regress toward the mean. Whenever possible, it is best to use groups of subjects whose responses cover the entire range of possible scores and to avoid relying on groups with extreme scores.

Selection. The results of studies not employing random selection may be biased by the sample selection. For example, if the first five people who volunteer to participate in a study are assigned to an experimental group and five who refuse are assigned to a control group, there is not a way to insure comparability of groups. Those who volunteered to participate in the study are clearly different. Randomization should be employed whenever possible to insure group homogeneity.

Mortality. One can expect that not all subjects will finish an experiment. If different numbers of subjects in different experimental groups "drop out," the consequence is unequal group size and the possibility that those remaining differ from the population as a whole. When mortality of subjects is an issue, attempts to equalize the groups might be made by randomly dropping subjects, adding subjects, or employing a statistical correction such as using the group mean to represent the scores of the "dropouts." The dropout rate, especially if it is high, should be reported and explained.

Interactions with Selection. Many factors can interact. Suppose that an investigator's intent was to compare socioeconomic groups in their responses to a patient education program. If the groups are not comparable in terms of other variables such as age, sex, and educational level, differences may result that are not due solely to socioeconomic group.

Diffusion of Treatment. This occurs when members of the control group learn about the experimental intervention. The control group, as a consequence, may behave not as a control group but more as an experimental group. Therefore, differences between the control group and experimental group will not be easily discernible. The researcher should attempt to keep the two groups separated to control the sharing of information between them.

Compensatory Equalization of Treatments. This is similar to diffusion of treatment, occurring when those selected to be controls are subjected to special circumstances, causing them to behave more like the experimental groups. Suppose that in a large-scale experiment to evaluate primary nursing several hospital units were randomly selected to institute various modifications of a primary nursing approach to patient care. The units not chosen—the control units—may hire more staff or may structure assignments differently, causing their units to be very similar to the primary nursing units.

Compensatory Rivalry. There are some experimental situations in which the nature of experimental interventions must be made public, generating rivalry between the experimental and control groups. In the previous example it is very likely that the control units, those without primary nursing, would compete with the experimental units.

Demoralization Effects. Instead of rivalry between experimental and control groups, those in the control group may become less motivated and not work as hard as normal. This will cause the differences between the experimental and control groups to be amplified.

Local History. The effects of local history may affect results when testing conditions for groups are dissimilar. If subjects in an experimental group are tested at one time and place and subjects in the control group at another time and place, it may be difficult to demonstrate that environmental conditions or an outside event did not bias results. Therefore every attempt must be made to create constant testing conditions.

External Validity

Although true experimental designs are able to control for many threats to internal validity, controlling threats to external validity is not as easy. External validity is concerned with generalizability of findings and is defined as the extent to which results of a study are applicable to other people or settings. Other factors must be considered. Huck, Cormier, and Bounds (1974) have described two components of external validity: population validity, concerned with the generalization of results to other subjects, and ecological validity, concerned with the generalization of results to other settings. As shown in Table 6–2, there are eleven threats to external validity; two are specific to population validity and nine to ecological validity. Again, please note that many of the sources of external invalidity are not a function of inadequate design but are factors associated with

Table 6–2. THREATS TO EXTERNAL VALIDITY

Population
Experimentally accessible population
Interaction of treatment effects with subject variables
Ecological
Describing the independent variable
Describing and measuring the dependent variable
Multiple-treatment interference
Interaction of the experimental treatment and history
Interaction of the experimental treatment and time
Sensitization to measurements
Hawthorne effect
Experimenter effect
Novelty of the experiment

people (either the experimenter or subjects) and how they influence the experimental situation.

Experimentally Accessible Population Versus Target Population. Theoretically, random selection from a defined population insures that generalizations can be made to that population. The sample is then representative. Random assignment is not quite the same thing, as will be discussed later. When random assignment is used, all subjects who meet predetermined criteria are admitted into a study and then randomly assigned to experimental or control conditions. As a consequence generalizability is limited to only those subjects studied. With random assignment the population cannot be greater than the subjects who are accessible to the experimenter.

Interaction Between Treatment and Subject Characteristics. Another threat to external validity is the possible interaction between characteristics of the subjects and treatment. To illustrate, in a study of the influence of exercise on the cardiovascular system, a certain type of exercise may be more readily performed by those who have an athletic history, are male, are of a certain body build, are of a certain age group, or are of normal weight. A researcher not aware of such interactions may wrongly assume that one kind of exercise is appropriate for all subjects.

Describing the Independent Variable. External validity is jeopardized when the independent (manipulated) variable is not adequately described. The experimental procedures and activities as well as the length of time used in treatment must be described so that it is clear just what is to be generalized. Too often the methods section of a research report is so vague that others are left puzzled as to what variables were manipulated and how the manipulation was done. A good rule of thumb is that the procedures associated with the independent variable should be presented in sufficient detail so that the reader can, if desired, replicate the experimental intervention.

Describing and Measuring the Dependent Variable. Like the independent variable, the dependent (outcome) variable must also be clearly described. Suppose the dependent variable in a particular study is level of anxiety. The researcher must operationally define anxiety and describe how anxiety was measured and quantified. The measuring instrument must have demonstrated reliability and validity and be quantified and analyzed using correct measurement and statistical procedures under comparable circumstances.

Multiple-Treatment Interference. This threat to external validity occurs when more than one experimental treatment is used with the same subjects. While the effects of the first treatment may be readily discernible, the results of the second are confounded by the first. Thus it is impossible to determine the extent of the influence of the second treatment. As the number of experimental treatments increases, the complexities of the problem accelerate.

Interaction of History and the Treatment Effect. Events occurring at the time a study is conducted may interact with the effects of the experimental treatment. It is possible that concurrent events can cloud the results in such a way that similar results would not be possible on another occasion. The results of a corporate exercise study, for example, might be influenced by the fact that a company executive recently suffered a myocardial infarction. If the study were conducted at another time, employees may not participate with the same intensity, and outcomes would be quite different.

Interaction of Time of Measurement and Treatment Effects. In the usual situation the effects of an experimental treatment are measured immediately following the treatment. If, however, the treatment effects do not occur immediately, a researcher may conclude that the treatment was not effective. The reverse is also true. If the results of an experimental intervention do occur immediately but dissipate over time and measurements are not immediate, a researcher may also arrive at erroneous conclusions. One way to guard against this threat to external validity is to take multiple measures of the dependent variable following the experimental treatment.

Pre-Test and Post-Test Sensitization. A pre-test can confound the results of the experimental treatment by sensitizing subjects to the expectations of an experiment. Pre-test sensitization often occurs when attitude or opinion measures, personality tests, and interviews are used prior to an intervention. The length of time between a pre-test and an experimental treatment can also be an issue. It is quite possible that the results of an experiment are somewhat dependent on a post-test, particularly one that gives clues to facilitate recall of experimental procedures or facts that will cause subjects to respond in a certain way.

Hawthorne Effect. When subjects are aware that they are participating in a study, several factors may operate. Cues in the experiment that convey the investigator's intent to subjects may influence behavior. Subjects may also become apprehensive and anxious because of study participation. Subjects may want to be good subjects and perform the way they perceive the researcher would like because they know their performance will be evaluated. Finally, subjects may believe in the effectiveness of the experimental treatment because it is part of a scientific experiment. All of these factors are unrelated to the experimental treatment, but may bias the outcomes of the treatment.

Novelty and Disruption Effects. The novelty of an experimental situation may prove more influential than an experimental treatment. This is particularly the case where new and innovative programs are being tested. A swimming program aimed at decreasing depression in psychiatric patients may prove more novel than the usual running program instituted years before. A novel experimental intervention may be initially disruptive until both researcher and subjects feel comfortable with the experimental procedures. This is why it may be wise to allow time for subjects to become familiar with the research protocol so that results will not be influenced by feelings of discomfort or difficulty adapting to procedures.

Experimenter or Rosenthal Effect. Sometimes an experimenter may unknowingly influence how subjects respond to an experimental intervention. Verbal cues, behavioral cues, appearance, dress, age, sex, religious affiliation, and political preference may all communicate subtle cues to subjects and influence responses to the experimental treatment.

Specific Experimental Designs

The true experimental designs were defined by Campbell and Stanley (1966) to distinguish them from pre-experimental and quasi experimental designs. Table 6–3 lists the designs belonging to each of these three categories. Each design will be discussed and illustrated in accompanying figures. The following notation is used. The letter X is used to signify the independent or manipulated variable. The letter M is used to represent the time when a measurement is taken, with

Table 6–3. PRE-EXPERIMENTAL, EXPERIMENTAL, AND QUASI-EXPERIMENTAL DESIGNS

Pre-experimental	Quasi-experimental
One Shot Case Study	Time Series
One Group Before, After	Nonequivalent Control Group
Static Group Comparison	
Experimental	
Randomized Control Group Before, After	
Solomon Four Group	
Factorial	
Randomized Control Group After Only	

subscripts indicating sequence of measurement. Other design-specific notation is defined on the figures.

The three pre-experimental designs include the One Shot Case Study; the One Group Before, After design; and the Static Group design (Figures 6–1 to 6–3). When a One Shot Case Study (Figure 6–1) is used, an independent variable is introduced to a single group and a subsequent measurement is taken. This design allows a group to be studied only once and negates the importance of a comparison or control group.

The One Group Before, After design (Fig. 6–2) does incorporate two measurement periods, allowing one to derive some indication of the impact of the independent variable. However, it too is lacking a comparison or control group. The Static Group Design (Figure 6–3) does include an additional group as a source of comparison but suffers from the lack of pre-measures and randomization.

X	M_2

Let: X = the experimental treatment (independent variable)
M_2 = post-test of the dependent variable

Procedure:

1. Expose subjects to an experimental intervention, i.e., an independent variable
2. Measure the dependent variable following the intervention

Figure 6–1. One Shot Case Study (pre-experimental). (Adapted with permission from Donald T. Campbell and Julian C. Stanley: *Experimental and quasi-experimental designs for research*. Copyright 1963 by Houghton Mifflin Company.)

M_1	X	M_2

Let: X = independent variable (IV)
M_1 = pre-test
M_2 = post-test

Procedure:
1. Administer a pre-test of the dependent variable
2. Expose subjects to an experimental intervention, i.e., an independent variable
3. Administer a post-test of the dependent variable

Figure 6–2. One Group Before, After design (pre-experimental). (Adapted with permission from Donald T. Campbell and Julian C. Stanley: *Experimental and quasi-experimental designs for research*. Copyright 1963 by Houghton Mifflin Company.)

The true experimental designs (Figures 6–4 to 6–7) include the Randomized Control Group Before, After design; the Solomon Four Group design; the Factorial design; and the Randomized Control Group After Only design. Generally, experimental designs are considered the most powerful. Internal validity is upheld and it is generally possible to establish cause and effect, specifically that the introduction of an independent variable influenced changes in a dependent variable. The perfect experiment is one in which an independent variable is manipulated, randomization is employed, and a control group is used for comparison.

Group A	X	M_2
Group B	—	M_2

Let: X = independent variable
M_2 = post-test

Procedure:
1. Expose only group A to the experimental intervention (independent variable)
2. Administer a post-test of the dependent variable to both groups

Figure 6–3. Static Group design (pre-experimental). (Adapted with permission from Donald T. Campbell and Julian C. Stanley: *Experimental and quasi-experimental designs for research*. Copyright 1963 by Houghton Mifflin Company.)

The Randomized Control Group Before, After design (Figure 6–4) is often considered the workhorse of traditional experimentation. Both the experimental and control groups are randomly selected and only the experimental group is subjected to the experimental (independent) variable. If the experimental group differs significantly from the control group on the pre-test, a statistical adjustment can be made on the post-test scores of both groups using the analysis of covariance, a procedure to be discussed later. This design controls for factors that may jeopardize internal validity but is not as powerful as the Solomon Four Group design.

The Solomon Four Group design (Figure 6–5) controls not only for factors jeopardizing internal validity but for threats to external validity as well. It is an extension of the Randomized Control Group Before, After design, but note that the third and fourth groups are not initially measured and that the fourth group, in addition to not being measured upon entry into the study, is not exposed to the independent variable. This design controls for the biases of both the pre-test and the independent variable. The appropriate statistical procedure for data analysis for the Solomon design as well as the Factorial design is the analysis of variance.

Factorial designs are also considered experimental designs. As seen in Figure 6–6, this kind of design allows more than one independent variable to be evaluated. Subjects are randomly assigned to a treatment combination, and the effects of each treatment variable are assessed. This design can be extended to include more than two factors and can incorporate both a pre-test and a post-test. Such an approach was used by Fehring (1983), who employed a three-group experimental design to examine the effects of biofeedback-aided relaxation on the psychological stress symptoms of college students. Subjects were randomly assigned to one of three treatment conditions and had psychological stress symptoms measured before and after an eight-week experimental period. Thorough detailed explanations of the many variations of factorial designs are given in texts such as Kirk (1968).

The Randomized Control Group After Only design (Figure 6–7) is useful for situations in which a pre-test is not possible. The most critical element of this design is the fact that it avoids contaminating pre-test effects. It is essential, however, that randomization procedures be used to assign subjects to support the comparability of the groups. Without a pre-test or pre-measure, measuring change is not possible.

*E	M_1	X	M_2
*C	M_1		M_2

Let: X = independent variable
M_1 = pre-test
M_2 = post-test
E = experimental group
C = control group
* = randomization

Procedure:

1. Randomly select subjects from a defined population
2. Randomly assign subjects to a control or experimental group
3. Pre-test both groups
4. Expose the experimental group to the independent variable
5. Post-test both groups

Figure 6–4. Randomized Control Group Before, After design (experimental). (Adapted with permission from Donald T. Campbell and Julian C. Stanley: *Experimental and quasi-experimental designs for research*. Copyright 1963 by Houghton Mifflin Company.)

*Group A	M_1	X	M_2
*Group B	M_1		M_2
*Group C		X	M_2
*Group D			M_2

Let: X = independent variable
M_1 = pre-test
M_2 = post-test
* = randomization
Group A = pre-, post-test experimental group
Group B = pre-, post-test control group
Group C = post-test only experimental group
Group D = post-test control group

Procedure

1. Randomly select and randomly assign subjects to one of four groups
2. Pre-test Groups A, B
3. Expose Groups A, C to independent variable
4. Post-test all groups

Figure 6–5. Randomized Solomon Four Group design (experimental). (Adapted with permission from Donald T. Campbell and Julian C. Stanley: *Experimental and quasi-experimental designs for research*. Copyright 1963 by Houghton Mifflin Company.)

Teaching Interventions (X_2)

Time(X_1)	*Morning*	A	B	E
	Evening	C	D	F

Let: X_1 = time
X_2 = experimental interventions

Procedure:

1. Subjects assigned at random to one of the treatment combinations

Figure 6–6. Factorial design: three teaching interventions (X_2). (Adapted with permission from Donald T. Campbell and Julian C. Stanley: *Experimental and quasi-experimental designs for research*. Copyright 1963 by Houghton Mifflin Company.)

Quasi-experimental designs (Figures 6–8 and 6–9) look like an experiment but lack at least one of the essential ingredients (randomization, manipulation, and control). The Time Series design and the Nonequivalent Control Group design are the most common quasi-experimental designs. The distinguishing feature of the Time Series design (Figure 6–8) is that measurements are taken prior to and following the introduction of an independent variable. Variations in

*E	X	M_2
*C		M_2

Let: X = independent variable, i.e., the intervention
M_2 = post-test
E = experimental group
C = control group
* = randomization

Procedure:

1. Randomly select and randomly assign subjects to an experimental or control group
2. Administer or expose the experimental group to the intervention, i.e., the independent variable
3. Administer a post-test of the dependent variable to both groups

Figure 6–7. Randomized Control Group After Only design. (Adapted with permission from Donald T. Campbell and Julian C. Stanley: *Experimental and quasi-experimental designs for research*. Copyright 1963 by Houghton Mifflin Company.)

$$T_1 \quad T_2 \quad T_3 \quad X \quad T_4 \quad T_5 \quad T_6$$

Let: T = points in time at which dependent variable is measured
X = independent variable

Procedure:
1. Several measures of dependent variable are taken before and after introduction of the independent variable.

Figure 6–8. One Group Time Series design. (Adapted with permission from Donald T. Campbell and Julian C. Stanley: *Experimental and quasi-experimental designs for research*. Copyright 1963 by Houghton Mifflin Company.)

the design are obvious. More than one subject can be used, and as many measurements are taken as are deemed necessary.

Time series analysis is very useful when an equivalent control group is not available. Every individual is used as his or her own control. Differences between subjects and across time are easily assessed. Although this design resembles the one group design employing a pre-test and post-test of the dependent variable, the time series design has fewer problems of internal validity. To determine the physiological effects of bonding between humans and companion animals, a time series design was employed by a team of researchers

E	M_1	X	M_2
C	M_1		M_2

Let: X = independent variable
M_1 = pre-test
M_2 = post-test
E = experimental group
C = control group

Procedure:
1. Administer pre-test to both groups (note that it is not possible to randomize)
2. Expose the experimental group to the independent variable
3. Administer the post-test to both groups

Figure 6–9. Nonequivalent Control Group. (Adapted with permission from Donald T. Campbell and Julian C. Stanley: *Experimental and quasi-experimental designs for research*. Copyright 1963 by Houghton Mifflin Company.)

(Baun and colleagues, 1984). Blood pressure, heart rate, and respiratory rate were recorded at baseline until stabilization occurred. The experimental intervention, that of petting a dog, was then introduced. Post measures were taken at three-minute intervals for nine minutes.

The Nonequivalent Control Group design (Figure 6–9) is useful when it is not possible to assign subjects randomly to experimental and control groups. The groups are naturally assembled collectives, such as patients on two different hospital units. While it is not possible to assign subjects randomly to groups, it is possible to determine randomly which group receives the experimental treatment. The Nonequivalent Control Group design is more powerful when it is demonstrated that the two groups perform in a similar way on the pre-test.

SINGLE-SUBJECT RESEARCH

Studies can be designed to look at only one subject from either a descriptive stance (case study) or experimental stance (single-subject experiment). The benefits of taking a single-subject approach are numerous. Thus, it is perplexing that those involved in nursing research have been reluctant to recognize single-subject approaches as legitimate research. Yet the research productivity of other disciplines such as clinical psychology, medicine, and psychopharmacology flourishes because they recognize the contributions to professional knowledge that are made with N = 1.

Single-subject research does not require huge numbers of subjects and can be carried out in any setting. One individual can be studied intensively, and his or her responses are not masked as they would be if they became part of grouped data.

The critics of single-subject research say that the results from such studies cannot be generalized to others. This is not entirely true, as one might expect that results obtained from one individual will more than likely be obtained from another similar individual. However, it is only through replication of the study with similar subjects that the generalizability of results will be supported.

OTHER RESEARCH APPROACHES

Several other research approaches bear mentioning. If they seem to be very similar to designs you have just read about, it is because many of them are. There is considerable overlap in design terminology, and many times some design experts make fine distinctions between designs or research approaches not made by others. Furthermore, nurse researchers adopt many designs and approaches from various disciplines where similar approaches are labeled in differing ways.

Ex Post Facto. An ex post facto design is one in which there is no control over variables because they have already occurred. An ex post facto approach might be taken to study pre-menopausal physical activity patterns of post-menopausal women. Note that the researcher cannot control these physical activity patterns because they have occurred prior to the study.

Laboratory Experiment. In a laboratory experiment all possible sources of contamination are kept to a minimum. Just as the name implies, a laboratory experiment is conducted in a controlled environment apart from usual day to day activities. Just as in any experiment, one or more independent variables are manipulated.

Field Experiment. A field experiment is carried out in a realistic setting. This approach is similar to a laboratory experiment, with the primary difference being the degree of control.

Retrospective Study. Here past events and factors are examined to explain a current event or disease. A group with heart disease, for instance, may be examined, and then factors occurring in the past may be traced that could help explain occurrence of the disease.

Prospective Study. Unlike a retrospective study, a prospective study is initiated to uncover factors associated with a disease or event from the present time forward. Thus a prospective study is longitudinal. From an epidemiological standpoint, such an approach determines the prevalence of a disease at the onset of a study and compares this information with information obtained at specific future time periods.

Cross-Sectional Study. Most researcher designs are cross-sectional, meaning that they are one-time studies of a defined population at a specific time period. Although many times a longitudinal approach would provide more valuable information, a cross-sectional approach is taken because it is the most realistic in terms of time, people, money, and resources.

Longitudinal Study. A longitudinal study is one in which subjects are followed for a specified time period. Initially base line measurements are taken, and the measurements are repeated at specified intervals.

SELECTING A DESIGN

Of primary concern is whether the design is appropriate for the research question. Astute researchers realize that design problems can result in meaningless data. Practical considerations are also important. Availability of research facilities, such as computers and duplicating equipment, availability of appropriate clinical sites, and budgetary constraints are factors that often lead an investigator to select design alternatives that may be more convenient and economical.

There may also be unique aspects of the setting, clinical or otherwise, that may introduce unplanned circumstances requiring changes or modifications in one or more aspects of the research design. It cannot be emphasized enough, therefore, that designs are selected and applied on a tentative basis. An original research plan must be open to change.

ELEMENTS FOR CRITIQUE OF A RESEARCH DESIGN

- Is the design clearly indicated?
- Is it appropriate to the problem?
- Is there sufficient knowledge of the problem to warrant the design?
- Does the design control for or minimize the extraneous variables that may affect the results of the study?
- How does the design control for threats to internal or external validity?
- What modifications, if any, could be made in the research design to improve it without significantly increasing the time and money required to carry out the study?
- Will it be possible for other researchers to replicate the research design of the study?

Questions and Activities

1. *Of all the threats to internal validity, which would you say is the most critical? Support your answer.*
2. *If cold weather is highly correlated with the number of coronary admissions to an emergency room, what factors would preclude one from declaring that cold weather causes myocardial infarction?*
3. *What kinds of studies are amenable to correlational design? Experimental design?*
4. *Under what circumstances would a quasi-experimental approach be preferred?*
5. *Discuss the factors involved in selecting a design for a study.*
6. *Discuss the notion that external validity is worthless without internal validity.*

Bibliography

Baun, M.M., Bergstrom, N., Langston, N. F., and Thoma, L. (1984). Physiological effects of human/companion animal bonding. *Nursing Research, 33*(3), 126–129.

Campbell, D.T., and Stanley, J. C. (1966). *Experimental and quasi-experimental designs for research.* Chicago: Rand McNally.

Cook, T.D., and Campbell, D.T. (1979). *Quasi-experimentation: Design and analysis issues for field settings.* Chicago: Rand McNally.

Diers, D. (1979). *Research in Nursing Practice.* Philadelphia: J. B. Lippincott.

Donahue, M.P. (1983). Isabel Maitland Stewart's philosophy of education. *Nursing Research, 32*(3), 140–145.

Dukes, W.F. (1965). N = 1. *Psychological Bulletin, 64,* 74–79.

Duxbury, M.L., Armstrong, G.D., Drew, D.J., and Henly, S.J. (1984). Head nurse leadership style with staff nurse burnout and job satisfaction in neonatal intensive care units. *Nursing Research, 33*(2), 97–101.

Fehring, R. (1983). Effects of biofeedback-aided relaxation on the psychological stress symptoms of college students. *Nursing Research, 32*(6), 362–366.

Holm, K. (1983). Single subject research. *Nursing Research, 32*(4), 253–255.

Huck, S.W., Cormier, W.H., and Bounds, W.G., Jr. (1974). *Reading statistics and research.* New York: Harper and Row.

Kirk, R.E. (1968). *Experimental design: Procedures for the behavioral sciences.* Belmont, CA: Brooks-Cole.

Kirchhoff, K.T. (1982). A diffusion survey of coronary precautions. *Nursing Research, 31*(4), 196–201.
Stern, P.N. (1978). Stepfather families: Integration around child discipline. *Issues in Mental Health Nursing 1*(2), 50–56.
Stern, P.N. (1980). Grounded theory methodology: Its uses and processes. *Image. 12*(1) 20–23.
Waltz, C., and Bausell, R. B. (1981). *Nursing Research: Design statistics and computer analysis.* Philadelphia: F.A. Davis.

IMPLEMENTING A RESEARCH STUDY

This unit begins with a discussion of the characteristics of data collection instruments and their design and selection. Specific data collection techniques such as observation, scaling, and interviews are described. An important element in data collection, the concept of measurement, is addressed in the chapter that follows. The unit concludes with a discussion of sampling, both probability and non-probability.

7

Locating, Designing, and Using Research Instruments

OBJECTIVES

After completing this chapter the reader will be able to:

1. Assess the utility of investigator-designed versus published instruments.
2. Describe sources for locating research instruments.
3. Describe the factors to consider in selecting a research instrument.
4. Differentiate between types of questionnaire items.
5. Describe factors to consider in question construction.
6. Examine factors involved in observation as a data collection method.
7. Discuss the use of interviews and questionnaires.
8. Describe commonly used scaling techniques.
9. Discuss the use of physiological measures in nursing research.

RESEARCH INSTRUMENTS

The old adage that something is "only as strong as its weakest link" is certainly relevant to research instruments, that is, the tools and measurement devices used to collect data of the study. The ultimate strength of a study and the validity of its conclusions are directly dependent upon the quality of the data collection instruments. Thus, the first sections of this chapter are devoted to a discussion of research instruments, their selection and development.

Published Instruments Versus Investigator-Designed Instruments

One of the first questions a researcher must consider when planning the collection of data is whether to use an established measuring device or to create a new and unique tool for use in the study. Advantages and disadvantages are evident with either choice, but there are a number of reasons why an existing instrument is preferable to use. First, use of a standardized measurement tool allows direct comparisons to be made to other studies. Thus, an individual study has improved generalizability and is more likely to add to the body of knowledge. An added benefit is that existing instruments are usually more economical, since construction of a new instrument can sometimes be quite costly. On the other hand, a self-constructed instrument can be made more specific to the research situation so that it is more precisely tailored to the particular questions and hypotheses of the study. However, given a choice between designing a new instrument or using one that has already been constructed, most experienced researchers would say, "Why reinvent the wheel?" and would probably advise using established and standardized instruments rather than risking use of a newly developed one. Thus, the search for existing instruments is often the first step in planning the methods of a study.

Locating Research Instruments

Though many research instruments are available to investigators, finding an appropriate tool that fits the design of a particular study can sometimes be like looking for a needle in the proverbial haystack. Fortunately, a number of resources are available to aid in the search. Some of them are described in the following paragraphs.

Reports of Previous Research. Analysis of previously conducted research of similar questions can often yield potential instruments. An imaginative search might include not only studies of similar or related constructs but perhaps studies on similar populations or studies that approach a question in a similar manner.

Published Listings. Indexes and catalogs of available instruments can be a good source. Most will not only refer you to instruments but will give you summary information about reliability, validity, costs, uses, and other aspects. Some compilations even include copies or examples of the instruments themselves. A representative listing of such guides to research instruments is given in Table 7–1.

Table 7–1. SELECTED PUBLISHED SOURCES OF RESEARCH INSTRUMENTS

Psychosocial

Buros, O. (1973). *Tests in print II.* Lincoln, NE: University of Nebraska Press.

Buros, O. (editor) (1978). *The eighth mental measurements yearbook.* Volumes 1 and 2. Lincoln, NE: University of Nebraska Press.

Goldman, B., and Busch, J. (1974). *Directory of unpublished experimental mental measures.* Volume 2. New York: Human Sciences Press. (Volume 1 is edited by Goldman and Saunders.)

Reeder, L. G., et al. (1976). *Handbook of scales and indices of health behavior.* Pacific Palisades, CA: Goodyear.

Ward, M., and Fetler, M. (editors) (1979). *Instruments for use in nursing education research.* Boulder, CO: Western Interstate Commission for Higher Education.

Ward, M., and Lindeman, C. (editors) (1979). *Instruments for use in nursing practice and other health care variables.* Volumes 1 and 2, *Health manpower references.* U.S. Department of Health, Education, and Welfare, Publication No. HRA 78–53. (Supt. of Documents, U.S. Government Printing Office Stock No. 017–022–00628–6.) Appendix A has a listing of instrument compilation references.

Physiological

Cromwell, L., et al. (1980). *Biomedical instrumentation and measurements.* 2nd edition. Englewood Cliffs, NJ: Prentice-Hall.

Geddes, L. A., and Baker, L. E. (1975). *Principles of applied biomedical instrumentation.* New York: John Wiley & Sons.

Greenfield, N. S., and Sternbach, R. A. (1972). *Handbook of psychophysiology.* New York: Holt, Rinehart, and Winston.

Thomas, H. E. (1974). *Handbook of biomedical instrumentation and measurement.* Reston, VA: Reston.

Advice of Experts. Talking to experts in the field can often yield useful instruments and can save a researcher valuable time by avoiding a costly search of the literature. Experienced researchers are usually very willing to share their advice with beginning researchers. In addition, they may sometimes know of instruments in the process of development or of completed studies of instruments that have not yet been published (a process that is now sometimes as long as 4 or 5 years in some disciplines).

Serendipity. Serendipity refers to making a discovery by accident. Sometimes a researcher discovers an instrument unexpectedly when exploring another area of research. These fortuitous finds are rare but welcomed!

Selecting Research Instruments

When the search for an instrument has yielded a possibility, then the instrument must be critically evaluated. Is it a good choice for a particular study or should the researcher find another or construct a new one? Utilization of an existing instrument is contingent upon the answers to a number of questions. These considerations are summarized in Figure 7–1 and described in the following paragraphs.

Does the Instrument Match the Research Questions and Hypotheses? If the central purpose of the instrument is to allow the investigator to collect data relevant to the question under study, then an instrument that does not do so is useless. A researcher wants an instrument that will allow the gathering of data relevant to the question and that will test the relationships stated in the hypotheses. One can discover the greatest instrument in the world, with strong validity and reliability, good utility, and low cost, but if it does not address the problem under study, it is useless.

For example, suppose a researcher wants to study the physiological effects of anxiety on hospitalized patients. She might consider using the State-Trait Anxiety Inventory (STAI), a questionnaire that has been successfully employed in numerous studies of anxiety. However, she would be making the mistake of measuring the wrong aspect of the variable under study, because the STAI addresses the psychological aspect of the concept of anxiety. To study the physiological aspects of anxiety, as is planned in the research questions, the researcher would be wiser to turn to instruments that more directly measure physiological parameters, such as an electrocardiogram or sphygmomanometer.

Does the Instrument Measure Data at the Appropriate Level of Measurement for the Research Question? Determine the level of measurement of an instrument. (Refer to Chapter 8.) Is it nominal, ordinal, interval, or ratio? The answer to this question may have implications for the type of statistics that can be used to test the hypotheses of the study. If the instrument yields nominal level data, it will limit statistical testing.

What is the Risk to the Study Subjects in Using This Instrument? Psychological risks as well as physical risks must be taken into

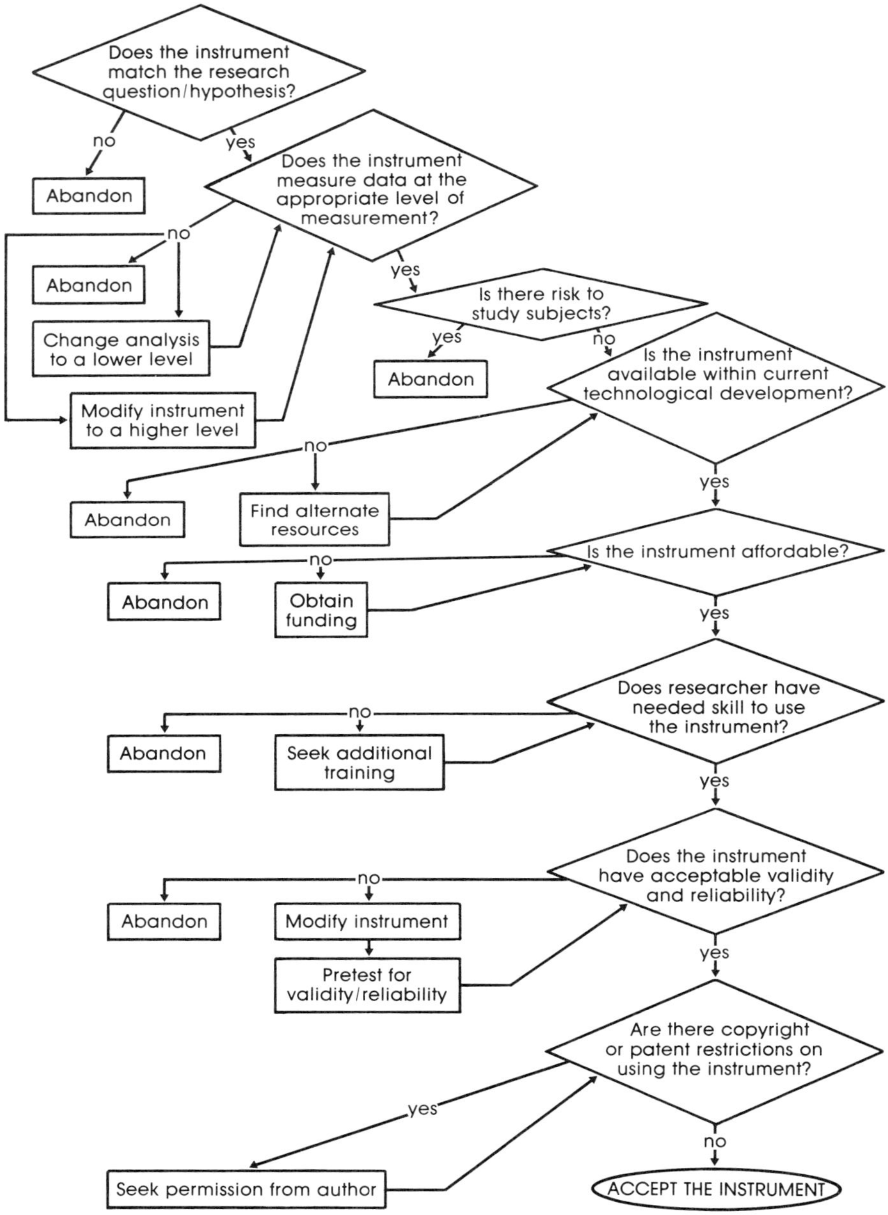

Figure 7–1. Flow diagram for assessing the utility of a research instrument.

account when deciding whether or not to use an instrument. If questions asked on an instrument are likely to significantly increase a subject's anxiety or if a survey is so lengthy as to tire a seriously ill patient, then the risk-benefit ratio must be carefully weighed, and an otherwise suitable instrument may be deemed inappropriate for the study.

Is the Instrument Available Within the Current State of Technological Development? The technology may not be available within your setting to use certain types of instruments, especially if they rely upon technological support. For example, it is common for many of the scales and questionnaires to require computer scoring and weighting of items. If the needed hardware or software programs are not accessible to the researcher, then those instruments may not be usable in that setting.

Is the Cost of the Instrument Warranted? The cost of an instrument can include such factors as fees paid for use of the instrument itself, outlay of resources required for materials related to administration or scoring of the instrument, costs related to training required to administer or interpret the instrument, or other hidden costs.

Is the Level of Skill Needed to Apply a Specific Instrument Appropriate to the Researcher's Preparation and Ability to Use the Instrument? Often the reliability and validity of an instrument are dependent upon specialized training required of the person administering the instrument. For example, most novices could probably administer a Rorschach test, but the interpretation of the results would be highly dependent upon the psychiatric skills and abilities of the practitioner.

Does the Instrument Have Established Validity and Reliability? The reliability and validity of an instrument are germane to its use. No matter how attractive an instrument may appear, if it does not measure what it was meant to measure (validity), or if it does not consistently measure the variable under question (reliability), it is of limited use in a study.

It is important to know the method used to establish reliability and validity of the tool, including the population on which it was tested. Is the population comparable to the one of the proposed study? Many times, scales and questionnaires are initially tested on college students, members of the military, or other normal groups.

When such is the case, the results obtained cannot necessarily be transferred to specific populations of patients. (In these situations the reliability and validity of the instrument must be re-established via a pilot test on the specified population.)

It is also wise to critically review the studies in which validity and reliability were tested. Were the methods sound? Does the strength of the findings warrant further use of the instrument? An added benefit is that problems with the tool are sometimes discovered.

Are There Copyright or Patent Restrictions on Using a Particular Instrument? In many cases, researchers are delighted to allow other investigators to use their tools, provided that the results are shared. It is in this way that a researcher can obtain larger and larger samples on which to base generalizations regarding validity and reliability of instruments. Another factor that may enter into a researcher's willingness to allow use of an instrument relates to his or her desire to make sure that there are quality controls on the use of the instrument. They may want to make sure that the instrument is used for its original intended purpose or that it is used by individuals who are going to be adequately trained in its proper use. In any event, courtesy demands a letter to the creator of the instrument requesting permission for its use.

In other cases, the use of an instrument is more restricted. Sometimes researchers seek to gain a profit from an instrument or they may merely charge a fee to recover costs of instrument development, which in many cases can be expensive. In this event, a researcher pays a fee, either to purchase copies of the instrument itself or to purchase scoring or administration devices.

If the answers to the above questions are favorable, then it is preferable to use an established instrument. Sometimes, however, a compromise approach may be taken whereby an established instrument is modified for a more specific use. This is a highly acceptable approach to take, provided that the appropriate permission is obtained from the original author.

CONSTRUCTING AN INSTRUMENT (QUESTIONNAIRE, SURVEY, INTERVIEW SCHEDULE)

Murphy's Law of Questionnaire Design: "Anything that can possibly be misunderstood in a questionnaire will be."

Instrument construction is a difficult, time-consuming, and sometimes frustrating endeavor. However, it is also a challenge and can be an outlet for creativity and thus can be a satisfying experience. Design of a survey or questionnaire is a skill that is broadly useful to health professionals, not only for those who are conducting research. It is inevitable that one will need to evaluate a program, survey a staff or patient population, or write test questions for students or patients, so the principles of instrument design can be applied broadly.

Types of Questions

Open-Ended Questions. Open-ended questions, also sometimes called free answer format, are those in which the respondent is asked to provide his or her own answer. This type of construction is most useful under the following circumstances:

1. *When the study is exploratory in nature.* Pilot studies often fall into this category. If a researcher is at the stage of generating questions or hypotheses, she may unknowingly lead respondents in a particular direction if she constructs the question responses. On the other hand, an open format will allow subjects to freely explore an issue or particular dimensions of a question without undue influence by the investigator.
2. *When the study aims at expansion of ideas.* When the purpose of the study is to introduce a subject, provide background for interpreting answers to other questions, solicit suggestions, obtain elaborations, evaluate arguments, or explore knowledge and memory, an open format is preferable.
3. *When the objectives of a study are at all ambiguous or if the topic under study is very complex.* When complex, multifaceted issues—ethical dilemmas, for example—are being explored, closed-ended responses cannot reflect the same richness of understanding as can open-ended ones. The difference is comparable to the contrast between a black-and-white and a color photograph.
4. *When the respondents vary greatly in their knowledge of the subject area.* For example, if one were studying hospital personnel's knowledge of acquired immune deficiency syndrome (AIDS), fixed responses understandable to physicians and nurses might be too complex for secretaries or other non-medical hospital workers.

In this case, an open format could be more effective. Similarly, if the reference point or knowledge level of the respondents is not known at all, an open structure is probably best.

5. *When the respondent is likely to have already formulated an opinion.* In the case of strong, previously held beliefs, question responses that are fixed may either not accurately reflect the subject's belief or otherwise bias the subject's response.

Open-ended questions are generally more difficult to analyze than fixed-format questions. In order to be qualified, the responses must be coded, and this can present a dilemma to the researcher, especially if a large or varied sample of subjects has responded. Another potential problem with open-ended questions is that the researcher may receive answers that are irrelevant to the research topic or do not directly address the question.

Closed-Ended Questions. Closed, or fixed alternative format, questions are those in which the investigator provides a set of responses and the respondent choses the one(s) that most closely match his or her own answers. This form is often preferred because there is greater uniformity of the responses and thus data analysis is expedited. Fixed format questions are more appropriate when:

1. *The researcher can anticipate the parameters of the question and of the respondents.* If the investigator knows the main dimensions of the issue, the range of possible responses, and the level of information and motivation in the population under study, a fixed format instrument is more easily constructed and will likely yield valid and reliable responses.
2. *The intent of the study is to divide subjects into groups.* If responses are to be measured, quantified, classified, or categorized, the task will be more readily accomplished with closed-ended responses.
3. *The respondents are poorly motivated to make the effort to formulate their own answers.* In these cases, the rate of response will probably be higher if the investigator provides the responses.

Closed-ended questions can be difficult to construct. One must be certain to provide all reasonably expected alternatives to the question without restricting the respondent. In other words, the list of alternative answers should be exhaustive while simultaneously being mutually exclusive.

Table 7–2. CHARACTERISTICS OF QUESTIONS

Positive	Negative
Clarity	Double-barreled
Exhaustive responses	Negative orientation
Mutually exclusive responses	Biased
Brevity	Complex
Applicability	Jargon-filled
Consistency	Sensitive
Objectivity	
Precision	

Construction of Questions

Writing questions for a questionnaire, test, survey, or interview schedule challenges even the most experienced researchers. Items that are clear to the researcher may not necessarily be understandable to the respondent. On the other hand, they may be clearly understood but totally misinterpreted. For this reason, pilot-testing with a sample similar to the one under study is essential. This section describes some positive and negative characteristics of questions. These are also summarized in Table 7–2.

Items should be as clear to the subjects as possible so that questions are not misconstrued. When questions are closed-ended, the researcher should make every effort to include all possible responses. Nothing is more frustrating to a subject than desiring to respond in a certain way and being forced to select the answer that is "closest," even though it is not the desired response. When exhaustive categories are not reasonably possible, an alternative is the use of an "other" choice. In this case, the researcher may also want to ask the respondent to specify what is meant by an "other" selection.

Table 7–3. CORRECT AND INCORRECT USE OF RESPONSE CATEGORIES

Incorrect	Correct
Overlapping responses	Mutually exclusive responses
______0 to 10 years	______0 to 10 years
______10 to 20 years	______11 to 20 years
______20 to 30 years	______21 years and older

Similarly, response categories should not overlap with one another. Table 7–3 illustrates the correct and incorrect use of response categories.

Questions should be kept as short and to the point as is possible without sacrificing clarity. Short items that can be read quickly have the best probability of yielding a high response rate. The length of individual questions as well as the total length of the questionnaire becomes especially significant when dealing with subjects who are physically or mentally compromised and who may tire easily.

The majority of items on a questionnaire should be relevant to most of the potential respondents. When a respondent encounters too many "not applicable" questions, he or she quickly loses interest in completing the remainder of the set.

If a question can be interpreted in a number of different ways, it is probably not precise. The way in which a question is asked should leave no doubt in the subject's mind exactly what information is desired. A useful technique to accomplish this is to include operational definitions with questions. For example, Table 7–4 illustrates how a question about alcohol consumption can be made more explicit by including a definition of what is meant by "a drink."

A number of things should be avoided in the construction of questions. For example, a double-barreled question (sometimes called a compound question) implies two separate responses. An example is an opinion poll that queries, "Do you favor abortion and gun control?" A respondent may support one but not the other and then is hard-pressed to give a single answer that accurately reflects his or her opinions.

Negatively worded items should also be avoided. Negative items leave a researcher open to the risk of misinterpretation. For example, a question stated as, "Do you agree or disagree that the American Hospital Association should not support prospective reimbursement for diagnosis-related groups?" could be misinterpreted because some people reading it quickly would overlook the "not." Even worse are double-negative questions such as, "Do you agree or disagree that few dying patients don't prefer to die at home?"

A question can also be leading or biased. A biased question has as its basis an erroneous assumption. An example is the comedic query, "When did you stop beating your wife?"

Table 7–4. EXAMPLE OF LAYOUT OF INSTRUCTIONS FOR A QUESTIONNAIRE

(Note that instructions to respondents are in italics to set them apart from the actual questions.)

SUBJECT INFORMATION SHEET

Identification Number ____________________ Date __________

The following information is needed for the statistical analysis of the results of this study. Please respond to the questions to the best of your ability. Circle only one answer for each question. Remember, all information will be kept completely confidential.

1. On an average night, how many hours do you usually sleep? *(Please circle one.)*
   Less than 6 hours in 24 1
   7 to 8 hours in 24 2
   9 or more hours in 24 3

2. Do you currently smoke cigarettes? *(Please circle one.)*
   Yes 1
   No *(If no, skip to question number 4.)* 2

3. Do you currently smoke: *(Please circle one.)*
   Less than 1 cirgarette per day 1
   Less than ½ pack per day 2
   Between ½ pack and 1 pack per day 3
   More than 1 pack per day 4

4. Do you ever drink alcoholic beverages? *(Please circle one.)*
   Yes 1
   No *(If no, skip to question number 6.)* 2

5. Do you currently drink: *(Please circle one.)*
   Less than 1 drink per week 1
   1 to 2 drinks per week 2
   3 to 6 drinks per week 3
   7 to 24 drinks per week 4
   25 or more drinks per week 5

(One drink = 12 ounces beer or 4 ounces wine or 1 ounce liquor)

Ordering of Questions

The recommended ordering or sequencing of questions is an area that remains somewhat controversial. There are a number of different methods in which to order items. If any one overall principle could be asserted, however, it would be that the order should be logical. Topics and questions should be arranged so that they make the most sense to the respondent. Similar questions should be grouped into units, and there should be a logical progression in the order of items in a unit and between units. Some of the various rationales are as follows (Table 7–5):

1. *Chronological:* If a researcher is requesting respondents to recall past events, it may be more logical to arrange items from the most recent past to the most distant past.
2. *General to specific:* The logic in this line of questioning is that if more general information is requested first, the respondent will not feel threatened as the researcher eases into questions of a more specific nature.
3. *Easy to hard:* A variation on the theme mentioned above, this ordering would present readily answered questions, such as demographic data, early in the questionnaire with the questions requiring more thought placed later.
4. *Least sensitive to most sensitive:* Particularly when one is assessing attitudes of a more sensitive nature, it makes sense to ask more neutral questions first so as not to inhibit later responses. If the most sensitive questions are asked first, some respondents may become intimidated and may choose not to complete the questionnaire.
5. *Most interesting to least interesting:* Some researchers are of the belief that starting a questionnaire with interesting and stimulating questions will engage the subject's interest and will motivate a respondent to finish the remaining questions. This approach,

Table 7–5. OPTIONS FOR THE ORDERING OF QUESTIONS ON A SURVEY

Chronological	Least sensitive to most sensitive
General to specific	Most interesting to least interesting
Easy to hard	

Table 7–6. EXAMPLE OF CONSISTENCY AND INCONSISTENCY OF THE FORMAT OF QUESTIONS

Consistent Format	Inconsistent Format
What is your sex?	Write in your sex. ________
☐ Male	Check your age. _____ under 30
☐ Female	_____ over 30
What is your age group?	Circle your marital status.
☐ Under 30	Single
☐ 30 and over	Married
What is your marital status?	
☐ Single	
☐ Married	

however, may be in conflict with some of the previously mentioned methods.

6. A final point to remember in ordering questions is that the answer to one question should not lead the respondent to a particular answer in a subsequent question.

Response Format

Several response formats are possible and the choice of format, although it may seem trivial, can make a big difference in the validity and reliability of data. Formats that permit (or even encourage) ambiguous responses should be avoided. Regardless of the format selected, it is important to be consistent and make the format the same for similar types of questions. Table 7–6 demonstrates both a consistent and an inconsistent response format.

Layout of the Questionnaire

The following are some general principles to consider in layout:

1. A questionnaire should have an attractive appearance. Maximizing white space on the form makes it appear uncluttered and less intimidating.
2. Avoid putting more than one question per line (the second one may be overlooked).

3. *Never* use abbreviations in questions.
4. Make sure the printing is in an appropriate size. For example, surveys given to elderly or diabetic patients might more appropriately be printed in larger than normal type.
5. Always have a title and clearly written instructions at the beginning of the questions. If more than one page, end each page with instructions to continue to the next page. At the end, state that this completes the questions and thank the respondent for his or her answers.
6. If instructions are included within the questions, they can be made to stand out be using italics. (Refer to the example in Table 7–4.)
7. Time will be saved in data analysis if the coding of data responses (that is, the values assigned to the categories of each variable) is included directly on the form, provided it does not become distracting to the respondent. (An example is shown in Table 7–4.)

Length of the Questionnaire

Finding the ideal length for a questionnaire can be difficult. One does not want the questionnaire to be too long or there is the possibility that the subject may become fatigued and fail to complete all of the questions. Worse yet, a subject may take one look at a lengthy questionnaire and not even make the attempt to complete it. Generally speaking, a questionnaire that takes longer than 20 to 25 minutes to complete will probably yield a lower response rate.

Interestingly, questionnaires that are too short may also result in a lower response rate. There is some feeling that subjects may view a too-short questionnaire as being "unimportant."

Above all, the researcher should be sensitive to the population being studied. If subjects are ill, tire easily, or are easily distracted, a shorter questionnaire is more appropriate.

DATA COLLECTION TECHNIQUES

Data collection refers to how information from the real world can be elicited, systematically recorded, and quantified. Data collection instruments are the tools used in the data collection process. In this chapter, some of the more common data collection techniques and methods will be described.

Observation

Observation is one of the most common methods used in nursing practice, and so it is logical that it is often the method chosen by nurse researchers. One reason that observation is so popular is that so many phenomena are amenable to observation. Examples are such things as characteristics and conditions of individuals, verbal and nonverbal communication behaviors, activities, attainment of skills, and environmental characteristics. In fact, some data are available *only* through direct observation.

There are a number of advantages to observation (Table 7–7). First, it has very broad applicability and can be useful in large numbers of situations. Secondly, it is a direct method of data collection. Because it is direct, many believe it produces more credible information; as the old saying goes, "seeing is believing." Finally, observation has the capacity to capture data with increased depth. Many more details and nuances can be observed than could possibly be described in narrative statements.

On the other hand, observation comes with several drawbacks. One of the most serious is that it is vulnerable to human perceptual errors. As humans, we unintentionally interject our own distortions and biases into everything that we observe. For example, we may read into a situation certain elements based upon our own past

Table 7–7. ADVANTAGES AND DISADVANTAGES OF OBSERVATION

Advantages	Disadvantages
Broad applicability	Vulnerable to human perceptual errors
Directness	Presence of observer causes behavioral distortions
Credibility	More costly than other methods
Increased depth of data	Instruments difficult to construct
	Potential for invasion of privacy

experiences. One way to safeguard against such distortions is to use multiple observers, using the logic that their individual biases would tend to cancel each other.

Another disadvantage of observation as a data collection method is that the presence of an observer may in itself cause behavioral distortions. When people know they are being watched, they change their behavior. This is sometimes called reactivity or the reactive measurement effect. Many researchers attempt to guard against this by making the observer unobtrusive in some way, such as by using one-way mirrors.

Other disadvantages to observation are: it is less time-efficient than other methods and therefore is more expensive; the instruments for observers are often cumbersome and difficult to construct; and there is sometimes the potential for violations of informed consent or of privacy and confidentiality when people are observed.

Types of Observation. Several observation techniques are available to the researcher. Observations can be structured or unstructured. Unstructured observations are of two types: participant observation and critical incidents. In participant observation, the researcher enters a group either as a member or as an observer, known or unknown, for the purpose of observing it. A major advantage of participant observation is that it tends to preserve the naturalness of the situation. In addition, the researcher actually participates in the situation, and this may help her to form hypotheses that she might not otherwise derive. For this reason, participant observation is valuable in exploratory work. A disadvantage of this method is that it may be difficult for the researcher to gain entrance into the group. The observer may be forced to relinquish her way of life temporarily. In addition, it may be difficult for the researcher to maintain objectivity, particularly if she becomes close to group members. Finally, the success of participant observation is very dependent upon personal characteristics of the observer and how well she is able to assimilate into the group without changing the group. Record keeping in participant observation is done by logs and/or field notes.

Another method of unstructured observation is the critical incident report, also called anecdotes. The idea behind critical incidents is that observations need be made only of those specific incidents that have been found to have a marked significance to the problem under study. It is similar to participant observation but more focused on behaviors of particular interest. This technique may be helpful as an exploratory method of deciding what is to be observed. However, several problems do exist with this method. First, it requires judgment about what is critical. Second, truly critical incidents occur infrequently. Finally, the apparently critical occurrence may be only the culmination of several important events or it may simply be a catalytic agent precipitating an action and not the primary determinant.

Other forms of observation fall into the structured category. The procedure for developing structured observational techniques involves (1) deciding when to observe, (2) devising a system for obtaining accurate records, and (3) training observers.

Deciding when to observe involves selection of a sampling method. Two types are commonly used: time sampling and event sampling. With time sampling, a universe of time is identified and a sampling design, either systematic or random, is utilized. Time sampling is usually more representative than event sampling. Event sampling involves selecting only events or occurrences of a given class. The three major advantages of event sampling are: (1) its inherent validity, (2) the fact that it offers continuity of behavior, and (3) the fact that it can capture events of interest that are infrequent.

Recording of observations in structured observational procedures may be accomplished in a number of ways. Categories and/or checklists are often used. Categories require operational definitions and should refer to behaviors that are mutually exclusive. The number of categories should be small, and the influence of the observer's inference should be kept at a moderate level by providing specific examples of behaviors. The sign system is a form of category checklist. It involves a listing of categories, and the observer identifies the frequency of particular behaviors on the list. Rating scales are also used to record observations. (An example of an observational rating scale may be found in Appendix D.) Rating scales can be used alone or as an extension of the category system.

A number of mechanical aids can be employed to assist in recording of observations. Videotaping is one such aid often used in nursing studies. It offers the advantage of permanency, and it can capture complex behaviors. Also, it is often easier to conceal a camera than a human observer, making it somewhat less intrusive (remembering, of course, that this is always done with the subject's consent). However, videorecording offers the disadvantages of complexity, inconvenience, and expense. In addition, it can record only one view of a situation and may thus give the observer a distorted impression.

The training of observers is critical. Much of the training of observers is similar to the training of interviewers, but there are a few unique points. It is ideal to have the observers participate in the development of the recording instruments because they may help to point out psychomotor limitations. They may also help to clarify categories. The observer usually does not need to know why he is observing, and it may be preferable for him not to know in order to minimize observer bias. Observers should be without cultural differences from the observed population. Interrater reliability must be achieved.

Interviews and Questionnaires

In this section, interviews and questionnaires will be treated together since they have many similarities, both involving direct questioning. The term "questionnaire" is usually used when the interview schedule is self-administered. A phone survey is a specialized case of the interview. Table 7–8 summarizes some of the differences between interviews, questionnaires, and phone surveys.

Uses. Interviews and questionnaires are used to obtain information that would be difficult, if not impossible, to gather by other means; for example, it would be very difficult to determine a person's attitudes or opinions without questioning him. Interviews can be used as an exploratory device to help identify variables and relations, to suggest hypotheses, and to guide other phases of research. In other studies, an interview or questionnaire may be the main instrument to measure the variables. Or, they can supplement other methods, for example to follow up unexpected results, validate other methods, or delve deeper into the motivations of respondents and their reasons for responding.

Types of Interviews

1. *Standardized* (also called structured or fixed interviews): the questions, sequence, and wording are fixed by the investigator.
2. *Nonstandardized* (also called unstructured or open): the inter-

Table 7–8. COMPARISON OF CHARACTERISTICS OF INTERVIEWS, QUESTIONNAIRES, AND PHONE SURVEYS

	Mailed Questionnaire	**Telephone Survey**	**Personal Interview**
Cost	Low	Low/medium	High
Convenience	Excellent	Fair	Low
Response rate	Low (less than 50%)	High	Highest
Quality of information	Fair	Good	Excellent
Geographic distribution of sample	May be very wide	May be wide	Usually clustered
Complexity of questions	May be complex	Must be simple	May be complex
Use of visual aids	Good	Impossible	Excellent
Control of response situation	Poor	Fair	Good
Overall reliability and validity	Good	Fair	Best
Appropriateness for sensitive topics	Good	Fair	Fair
Ability to probe	Poor	Good	Excellent

viewer has freedom to develop each interview in the most appropriate manner for the situation. She is not held to specific questions.

3. *Semistandardized:* The interviewer may be required to ask a number of specific major questions, but she may be permitted leeway to use alternate questions and/or probe as she chooses.
4. *Focused:* Similar to nonstandardized type in that no specific questions are asked but special attention is given to specific topics or ideas.
5. *Nondirective:* Commonly used in psychiatry. The subject can express feelings on topics without waiting to be questioned. The subject has complete freedom to discuss a topic without pressure from the interviewer.

Collecting Interview Data. The quality of interview data is very dependent upon the skill of the interviewer; thus, interviewer training becomes a crucial element in the research process. Interviewers must at all times be polite, non-judgmental, non-leading, and able to establish rapport with subjects. Sometimes interviews are conducted by phone.

Collecting Questionnaire Data. Questionnaires can either be self-administered (singly or in a group) or they can be mailed or personally delivered. When questionnaires are not personally delivered, the researcher must ensure that subjects actually complete the questions, otherwise known as ensuring a high response rate. Factors positively affecting the response rate include a short, attractive format, a letter (preferably under the sponsorship of a reputable source) explaining the importance of the survey, and avoidance of holidays. Sometimes inducements are used to get people to return surveys. The inducement is not always in the form of money; it might be a self-addressed envelope or some other convenience measure.

Just as important as the respondents are the people who did not respond to the survey. It is important to attempt to determine the key characteristics of this group as well in order to ensure that there has not been some sampling bias or self-selection into the study sample.

Researchers should attempt to make sure that questionnaires and interviews are always administered under similar conditions to all subjects. For example, if some subjects are given a shorter time period than others, if their environment is less conducive, or if their instructions have differed, then the reliability of the answers becomes questionable.

Scales

A scale consists of a series of questions in which the responses are graded or weighted in some way to reflect the magnitude or quantity of a variable. The techniques of psychometric scaling are beyond the scope of this book. However, some of the more common scales used in nursing research will be described.

Likert Scale. The Likert scale (also known as the Likert response pattern or summated ratings) is popular because it is relatively easy to construct and score. Items are rated along a continuum of some sort and ordinarily contain three to five categories to which varying degrees of intensity are attached. A numerical weight is given to each response, and these are added to arrive at a total score. Weighting is

Table 7–9. EXAMPLE OF A LIKERT SCALE

	Strongly disagree	Disagree	Neither agree nor disagree	Agree	Strongly agree
I enjoy being a nurse.	1	2	3	4	5

the process of assigning numerical values to each response. An example of a Likert scale is shown in Table 7–9. The higher the total score, the more the subject agrees with the attitude or possesses the variable in question. The response categories may vary; commonly used ones are importance (very important/not important), similarity (very similar/not at all similar), and utility (very useful/not at all useful).

Graphic Rating Scale. The graphic rating scale is one in which the variable is qualitatively scaled along a continuum and the subject makes a direct rating on the scale. It is also easy to construct and demonstrates the relationship of one category to another. However, the drawback is that subjects may be reluctant to mark either extreme, with the result that most scores are concentrated in the central categories. An example of a graphic rating scale is shown in Table 7–10.

Semantic Differential Scale. The semantic differential scale reflects a measure of the meaning of a psychological, social, and/or physical object and then evaluates its characteristics using a series of bipolar adjectives placed at the endpoints of a seven-point rating scale. An example of a semantic differential scale is shown in Table 7–11.

Thurstone Scale. The Thurstone Scale (also known as the equal-appearing interval scale) consists of a battery of statements, each with a specific scale value that denotes the intensity of each statement. The scale values are usually determined by a panel of judges. Re-

Table 7–10. EXAMPLE OF A GRAPHIC RATING SCALE

My pain is very severe.	My pain is bad.	My pain is average.	My pain is minimal.	I have no pain.
1	2	3	4	5

Table 7–11. EXAMPLE OF A SEMANTIC DIFFERENTIAL SCALE

								Primary Nurse								
Fair	:	7	:	6	:	5	:	4	:	3	:	2	:	1	:	Unfair
Important	:	7	:	6	:	5	:	4	:	3	:	2	:	1	:	Unimportant
Warm	:	7	:	6	:	5	:	4	:	3	:	2	:	1	:	Cold

spondents are asked to select two to five statements from the list that best reflect their ideas about the variable in question. The weights of the statements selected are usually averaged to determine the score. Although the Thurstone approach results in more meaningful scores, the battery and weighting of the statements is time-consuming and difficult to construct. An example of typical statements to elicit attitudes about death in the format of a Thurstone scale is shown in Table 7–12.

Bias in Scaling. A potential problem with scaling techniques is that subjects may respond to questions with a particular systematic bias. Several types of bias should be guarded against:

1. *Social desirability:* The tendency of some individuals to misrepresent their attitudes by giving answers that are consistent with prevailing social attitudes.
2. *Extreme responses:* Some people tend to answer with extreme opinions, rather than the middle-of-the-road alternatives.
3. *Acquiescence response set:* The tendency to agree with statements regardless of content.

Physiological Measures

More and more nurses are interested in studying physiological variables and are tackling the techniques necessary for such studies.

Table 7–12. EXAMPLE OF STATEMENTS FROM A THURSTONE SCALE EXAMINING ATTITUDES ABOUT DEATH AND DYING

Death is a natural process that is merely another aspect of the life cycle.
Suicide is an acceptable alternative in some situations.
Dying is painful.
A person should not be told if he has a terminal illness.

Bioinstrumentation offers several advantages to the researcher. First, physiologic methods are more objective than many other methods of measurement, since they do not often require human interpretation or judgment about the results. They also usually allow variables to be measured with increased precision and sensitivity over psychological and sociological instruments. Finally, the validity of bioinstrumentation is often stronger than that of other types of instruments.

These advantages, however, are achieved at a cost. Much of the equipment needed for biophysical studies is extremely costly and complex and requires specialized training and skills for its use. In addition, safety considerations are often a factor, since many of these measures require invasive or unpleasant techniques. Nurse researchers can overcome some of these obstacles through consultation with colleagues in the basic sciences who have more experience and training in the use of such instruments.

It should also be noted that there are reliability and validity concerns when physiological instruments are used. These include attention to precision and accuracy. An important precaution is ensuring proper calibration of equipment.

A wide variety of analytical and monitoring techniques are now available, some of which are relatively easy and convenient to use with patients in clinical settings. Table 7–13 summarizes some of the instruments and techniques that are used to study physiological variables and differentiates which are more accessible for use in clinical settings.

Questions and Activities

1. *What factors should be considered in selecting a research instrument?*
2. *Suppose you want to study maternal-infant bonding. How would you decide whether or not to construct your own instrument?*
3. *Under what conditions is it more appropriate to use open-ended as opposed to closed-ended questions?*
4. *Discuss the potential sources of observer bias and how each might be controlled.*
5. *Of the approaches to interviewing, which do you think would be most appropriate for a study of parental grief?*

Table 7–13. SUMMARY OF SELECTED BIOPHYSICAL MEASUREMENT TECHNIQUES

Variable	Instrument	Potential For Use In Clinical Research
Blood pressure		
Direct	Pressure transducer	Often readily accessible in critical care settings; more invasive and difficult to use in other settings.
Indirect	Standard sphygmomanometer	Readily available in clinical settings.
	Random zero sphygmomanometer*	Designed specifically for research, it minimizes observer bias. Easy to use in clinical settings.
	Automated sphygmomanometer	More costly, but easy to use. May have lower reliability than other methods.†
Heart rate and rhythm	Electrocardiograph	Readily available in clinical settings.
	Holter monitor‡	Though sometimes complex to interpret, this technique offers the advantage of obtaining measures during a subject's normal activities.
Arterial blood pH, CO_2 and O_2 concentrations	Blood gas analyzer	Often accessible in critical care settings; a standard laboratory technique.
Percent saturation of hemoglobin	Oximeter	Convenient to use in clinical settings.
Tidal volume	Spirometer	

Table continued on opposite page

Table 7–13. SUMMARY OF SELECTED BIOPHYSICAL MEASUREMENT TECHNIQUES *Continued*

Variable	Instrument	Potential For Use In Clinical Research
Peak flow	Respirometer	
Temperature		
Core	Thermometer	
Skin	Thermistor	
	Temperature band	
Electrical activity of the brain	Electroencephalogram	Expensive equipment; may be complex to interpret.
Skeletal muscle action potentials	Electromyogram	Equipment is expensive.
Electrical skin conductance	Galvanometer	
Alkalinity or acidity of body fluids	pH meter	A standard laboratory technique.
Visual acuity	Snellen eye examination chart	Convenient to use.
Color vision	Ichikawa color blindness test booklet	Requires standardized environmental lighting.
Subcutaneous fat	Skinfold caliper	Portable, convenient to use.
Joint flexibility	Goniometer	Easily used to measure range of motion in most joints.
Muscle strength	Dynamometer	Noninvasive technique for evaluating muscle fatigue and/or strength.

*Wright, B. M., and Dore, C. F. (1970). A random-zero sphygmomanometer. *Lancet, 1*, 337–338.

†LaBarthe, D. R., Hawkins, C. M., and Remington, R. D. (1973). Evaluation of performance of selected devices for measuring blood pressure. *American Journal of Cardiology, 32*, 546–553.

‡Haughey, B. P. (1983). Holter monitoring: A method for nursing research. *Nursing Research, 32*(1), 59–60.

ELEMENTS FOR CRITIQUE OF RESEARCH INSTRUMENTS

- Are the data collection instruments clearly described?
- Was adequate rationale given for instrument selection?
- Were the instruments appropriate measures of the variables under study?
- Do the instruments measure data at the appropriate level of measurement?
- Is there evidence of satisfactory validity and reliability?
- Are validity and reliability reassessed for the specific population under study?
- Are the instruments pre-tested?
- Are the instruments consistent with the abilities of the subjects?
- Is there evidence that research personnel were trained in the use of the instruments?
- Is the time required for administration of the instrument realistic?
- Were the instruments administered in the same way to all subjects?
- Are the limitations of the instruments addressed?

Bibliography

Corbett, J. V. (1982). *Laboratory tests in nursing practice.* Norwalk, CT: Appleton-Century-Crofts.

Jagger, J. (1982). Data collection instruments: Sidestepping the pitfalls. *Nurse Educator*, May–June, 25–28.

Kerlinger, F. N. (1973). *Foundations of behavioral research.* 2nd edition. New York: Holt, Rinehart, and Winston.

Nunnally, J.C. (1978). *Psychometric theory.* New York: McGraw-Hill.

Orlich, D. C. (1978). *Designing sensible surveys.* Pleasantville, NY: Redgrave.

Sudman, S., and Bradburn, N. M. (1982). *Asking questions: A practical guide to questionnaire design.* San Francisco: Jossey-Bass.

Vredevoe, D. L. (1972). Nursing research involving physiological mechanisms: Definitions of the variables. *Nursing Research, 21*, 68–72.

Wooley, A. S. (1984). Questioning the mailed questionnaire as a valid instrument for research in nursing education. *Image, 16*(4), 115–119.

8

Measurement

OBJECTIVES

After completing this chapter the reader will be able to:

1. Discuss the concept of measurement.
2. Describe the levels of measurement.
3. Identify the role of measurement error in reliability assessment.
4. Enumerate approaches to reliability assessment.
5. Discuss approaches to the determination of validity.

Numbers and the operations associated with them are commonly understood. Scientists rely on numbers for communication of the magnitude of events or objects and the relationships between them. Measurement is the process whereby numbers are assigned to objects or events. Without measurement, scientific observations lose objectivity and precision. Measurement aims to provide a one-to-one correspondence between the variable measured and reality. When a measuring instrument succeeds in meeting this aim, it is said to be isomorphic, meaning that the numbers are not arbitrary but have a connection to reality. Because measurement allows phenomena to be described in numerical terms, hypotheses are more readily generated and statistics more easily applied. The ultimate test of measurement is how well it fosters scientific communication in numerical terms.

DEFINITION OF MEASUREMENT

The most frequently cited definition of measurement is "assigning numbers to objects according to rules" (Stevens, 1946). The popularity of this definition has not diminished with time. Taking the definition literally may be confusing. First of all, not everything is an object or event. Many psychosocial variables such as fear, anxiety, or alienation are too abstract to be seen or touched. Second, even when we can see or touch the object we intend to measure, we measure only attributes or properties of the object. We can measure an individual's height, weight, blood pressure, degree of anxiety, or level of motivation but cannot measure the individual himself. The same holds true for inanimate objects. Measurements of a conference room table are reflective of properties of the table, specifically length, width, area, height, and weight.

A better definition of measurement is one that incorporates the notion of measuring properties or attributes of objects, people, or events. Because measurement involves abstraction, it might best be thought of as the process whereby attributes of objects, events, or people are linked to empirical indicants, such as numbers, according to a set of rules.

Rules imply an explicit statement of procedures. Sometimes the rules are obvious, such as using a yardstick to measure length or height. At other times the rules are not so obvious, as when measuring learning or psychological processes.

Table 8–1. CROSS-EXAMINING A MEASUREMENT

Would additional measurements by the same instrument agree?
Would agreement be better or worse if the time interval between repetitions were increased?
What if different instruments were used?
What environmental influences are present?
Do differences exist between data collectors?
Are biases present due to reference standards or calibrations?
What procedures were used to ensure validity and reliability?

Rules also imply standardization. When rules are unclear, a measure is not well standardized and an undesirable situation may follow, one in which measurements made by one person cannot be replicated by another.

If a particular measurement was part of a legal controversy, one of two things might occur. The contending parties might agree that the measurement was correct, or, if the parties could not agree, the uncertainty attached to the measurement would need to be established. Questions that might prove useful in the cross-examination of a measuring instrument are presented in Table 8–1. The importance of each of these questions will be apparent as you proceed through the remainder of this chapter.

LEVELS OF MEASUREMENT

There are at least four levels or, as they are sometimes known, scales of measurement. They are presented in Table 8–2. The first or lowest level is the *nominal* level. Measurement at this level is categorical, and numbers are assigned to code or label information. For example, patients might be classified as acute or nonacute. We might assign the numeral 1 to acute and 2 to nonacute. These numbers tell us nothing more than whether a patient belongs in the category of acute or nonacute. Technically, numbers representing categorical data should not be treated mathematically. Hence, the conclusions drawn from nominal data are limited. Nonquantitative statistical procedures such as percentages and frequencies may be used.

The next level is the *ordinal* level, where numbers symbolize a ranking according to a defined attribute or criterion. An ordinal scale

Table 8–2. MATHEMATICAL OPERATIONS AND LEVEL OF MEASUREMENT

Level	Operation
Nominal	Equal or not equal ($=$, $\neq$)
Ordinal	Equal, not equal, greater than, or less than ($=$, $\neq$, $>$, $<$)
Interval	Equal, not equal, greater than, less than, addition, subtraction ($=$, $\neq$, $>$, $<$, $+$, $-$)
Ratio	Proportions in addition to all the interval operations

might be used to rank patients in terms of activity of daily living as shown in Table 8–3. While we can assign a rank order to patients on such a scale, we can never really know if completely independent is two times better than completely dependent; in other words, we do not know the distance between points on this scale. Purists have argued that the more powerful parametric statistics are not appropriate for ordinal data. But because the majority of psychosocial measures are ordinal, investigators have ignored this assumption to subject data to more powerful statistical tests.

At the *interval* level of measurement the distance between points on the scale is known. Fahrenheit temperature is an example of interval level measurement. Here zero is not absolute as is true of the *ratio* level of measurement, in which zero signifies the absence of the specific variable measured. The interval and ratio levels are the highest levels of measurement. The distinction between the interval and ratio level of measurement, namely the presence or absence of an absolute zero, is often a matter of how one interprets absolute zero. In nursing research it usually is not necessary to differentiate between interval and ratio measurement, as both levels employ the same statistical tests.

Mathematical operations theoretically meaningful for each meas-

Table 8–3. AN EXAMPLE OF AN ORDINAL SCALE

	Completely dependent				Completely independent
1. Bathing	1	2	3	4	5
2. Eating	1	2	3	4	5
3. Activity	1	2	3	4	5

urement level are shown in Table 8–2. Each level is cumulative, permitting additional mathematical operations as the level of measurement increases. At the nominal or categorical level, people or objects either belong or do not belong in a category. Patients can be labeled anxious or not anxious; the temperature of a liquid can be described as being hot or cold. At the ordinal level we can speak of greater than or less than. Patient A can be said to be more anxious than patient C, but less anxious than patient B. When a variable is measured at the interval level, numbers can be added or subtracted. It makes sense at this level to add subjects' scores to arrive at a total. Arterial pressure, body temperature, and pulse are but three examples of technically pure interval variables encountered in clinical practice. Finally, at the ratio level of measurement, all mathematical operations are acceptable. Because there is controversy as to what is ordinal and what is interval, the ratio level is also influenced. For now it is best to say that when a variable is ratio, we can compare the proportionate extent to which one subject differs from another. Here it is meaningful to speak of twice or three times as many.

THEORETICAL NOTION OF MEASUREMENT ERROR

All measurement contains error, either systematic or random. Systematic error influences measurement in an orderly way and does not influence outcomes to the same extent as random error, which is more difficult to control.

Suppose a thermometer used to measure the temperature of fluid was off by two degrees. All measurements taken with the thermometer would vary by two degrees. This is an example of systematic error, in which all measurements are influenced in the same way.

Random error is not quite that simple. It is unorderly and many times is left unrecognized or unacknowledged. For example, if a rating scale is to be used by more than one investigator to rate the quality and quantity of sleep in hospitalized patients, not only are the potential sources of error numerous but they may also fluctuate. There will be errors associated with the investigators, the patients, the environment, and the rating scale itself.

Every attempt must be made to control error. Investigators are obligated to control the error they are able to control and to acknowledge the possibility of error that is beyond their control.

Theory of True and Error Scores

This model is the oldest conceptualization of measurement error. In this model, each observation made during a measurement process is viewed as having two additive parts, that which is true and that which is error. Error is defined as random and unrelated to the true score. The true score as defined by Thorndike (1982) is the average of infinite repeated measurements taken with the same measuring instrument. Many argue that the model is overly simplistic and is thus not a representation of reality. However, the model does delineate a number of relationships useful in the design and evaluation of measuring instruments.

Using the subscripts o, t, and e for observed score, true score, and error, respectively, the model assumptions are shown in Table 8–4.

RELIABILITY

Reliability refers to the consistency and stability of a measurement. To be reliable a measuring instrument must consistently measure the same thing. Reliability is said to be a prerequisite for validity as there is little chance of measuring what we say we are measuring if we can not measure it consistently. It is very important to realize that evidence for reliability is gathered from groups of people who are

Table 8–4. THEORY OF TRUE AND ERROR SCORES

1. Every measurement observation is the sum of a true component and an error component. In other words, $X_o = X_t + X_e$.
2. Error is independent of true score.
3. Error is completely random. Thus it follows that there may be as many errors in the negative direction as in the positive direction. Furthermore, error is normally distributed.
4. Individuals possess true characteristics that persist through time.

Table 8–5. RELIABILITY AND ERROR

Approach	Sources of Error
Test-retest	Response variability of subjects; differences in administration of the test; time factors (changes in what is measured over time)
Parallel forms	Individual items
Split-half	How the test is divided
Cronbach's alpha	Relatively little error; requires only one administration

representative of the population for whom the measurement is intended. If, for example, evidence for the reliability of a measure of denial is gathered from a group of acute cardiac patients, then more than likely the measure will prove reliable for other groups of acute cardiac patients.

Reliability is more than just a property of a particular measuring instrument. There are at least two other important factors that must be considered: the sample used to gain support for reliability and the conditions under which the support was obtained. In the example of the measure of denial in acute cardiac patients, such a measure may or may not prove reliable for patients with a chronic condition such as chronic renal failure.

Approaches to reliability can be classified as external (test-retest and parallel forms) or internal (split-half and Cronbach's alpha). These approaches are listed in Table 8–5. Each approach accounts for a different source of error.

Test-Retest

This commonly used approach is easiest to understand. When the test-retest method is employed, the results of two administrations of the same measuring instrument are compared. The two administrations are best separated by a two- to four-week period. While evidence for the stability of a measuring instrument can be supported by this method, there are limitations. Both low and high correlations that have little to do with the instrument may result. If what one is attempting to measure has changed, it is likely that the resulting correlation will be low; for example, fear or anxiety can be significantly altered by the passage of time, particularly with a long time interval between testing situations. Reactivity can also contribute to underestimates of reliability. During the first testing an individual may become sensitized to what is being measured and demonstrate changes that may be attributed to the fact that he or she was measured. If it is an attitude that is being measured, such as the likelihood of voting for a change in the process of delivery of nursing care, an individual who responded positively when first asked may experience a preference change due solely to exposure to the issues involved. In this case the resulting correlation coefficient will be low.

An overestimate of reliability due to memory is another problem with the test-retest method. What is likely to happen is that an individual remembers responses given at the first testing and simply repeats such responses at the second testing. Memory exerts a powerful influence even when an investigator separates the testing session with the recommended two- to four-week time interval. It is understandable why the usual criticism of the test-retest method is that it results in an overestimate of reliability.

Parallel Forms

The parallel forms method has been used primarily in an educational context. In this approach two forms or variations of the same instrument are administered to the same group of people at either the same time or on two different testing occasions. The two forms are designed so as to measure the same phenomenon and should not differ from each other in any systematic way. This is usually guaranteed by randomly selecting items from a pool of items developed for measuring the same thing. If one were interested in measuring comprehension of a dietary patient education program, the parallel forms approach to support reliability might be used. Questions could be developed reflecting the objectives of the program at the same level of difficulty. The questions then could be randomly selected to create two forms of the test. The tests could then be administered to the same group of patients and the correlation between the two tests would provide the estimate of reliability. While many may elect to administer the tests on the same day, some experts advise that the tests be given about two weeks apart. If tests are administered on the same day, it is wise to alter the order of administration randomly.

There are advantages to the parallel forms method. The first is that the two forms can be administered on one testing occasion or on two occasions separated by approximately a two-week time span. Therefore the passage of time is not as great an issue as it is with the test-retest method. Another advantage is that the items on the two forms are different items, thus negating the error due to memory. If one were to criticize the parallel forms approach, it would have to be on the grounds that constructing two forms of a measuring instrument is often difficult and time-consuming and thus not practical in many measurement situations. In addition, it is not likely that two forms of a test could measure the phenomenon being studied in exactly the same way.

Split-Half Method

The split-half method can be conducted on one testing occasion. In this approach a total set of items is divided in half and comparisons are made between the two halves. The halves are often considered approximations to alternate forms. This method tends to underestimate reliability, as it is a known fact that longer tests are more reliable than shorter tests.

Because splitting the test in half can introduce bias, it is best to randomize the items into one half or the other. There is another equally important issue. When halves are correlated the obtained reliability coeffient is not reflective of the total test. However, a special procedure called the Spearman-Brown prophecy formula can be used to obtain an estimate of the reliability of the entire test.

Cronbach's Alpha

Another approach to reliability is that afforded by statistical procedures such as Cronbach's alpha, which is conceptually defined as the average of all possible split halves of a test. The value of this procedure is that only a single test administration is required. Furthermore, the obtained reliability coefficients are free from the problems encountered with other approaches, such as developing alternate forms, determining how to divide a test, or deciding how long to wait between testing intervals.

Cronbach's alpha can be derived from either a variance-covariance matrix or a correlation matrix. The correlation matrix approach to deriving alpha is more commonly used and can be explained as follows. First each item on a test is correlated with each of the remaining items. Then the average of the correlations is obtained and entered into the formula for Cronbach's alpha.

Alpha varies between 0.00 and 1.00 and in most situations provides a conservative estimate of the reliability of a test. An acceptable alpha for a new scale is 0.70 or above, and for a mature scale, 0.80 or above (Hinshaw and Atwood, 1982). The reliability of a test is only very rarely lower than alpha.

In conclusion, a reliability coefficient provides an index of the proportion of measurement that is considered true. Because of the nature of the reliability formulas, reliability will increase when additional items are added or as the spread or range of scores within a group increases.

VALIDITY

Validity is concerned with the extent to which a measuring instrument or test achieves certain aims. In other words, does the test measure what it claims to measure? Reliability is a prerequisite to validity, as a valid test must consistently measure the variable(s) it was designed to measure. Validity raises the question of "valid for what purposes?" Table 8–6 lists common approaches to validity and the purposes associated with each.

Table 8–6. APPROACHES TO VALIDITY

Content validity: observed and inferred based on item content.
Criterion-related validity: demonstrates a numerical association between the measured variable and an outside criterion.
Construct validity: uses statistics such as factor analysis to demonstrate the dimensions of a construct.

Content Validity

Content validity is concerned with the extent to which a test reflects the variable it seeks to measure. Content validity should be established when an instrument is developed. To ensure content validity the following steps are taken. First the variable to be measured is defined and relevant literature is examined to aid in delineating the variable's dimensions. The next step involves the construction of items that are representative of each dimension of the variable. At this stage it is better to construct too many rather than too few items, as items proving to be inadequate can later be deleted. Because there is no agreed-upon method for deciding the extent to which content validity has been achieved, the remaining step requires a judgment as to whether the items indeed reflect the defined variable and its dimensions. At this stage individuals who are familiar with the content area may be called upon to judge the appropriateness of the items.

Content validity is important for all tests but has particular implications for achievement and proficiency measures.

Criterion-Related Validity

This approach to validity requires relating scores on the test or measuring instrument in question to scores on an external criterion. The most critical element in criterion-related validity is the selection of a valid, reliable outside criterion. If the external criterion is not valid and reliable, the obtained validity coefficient has little credibility.

Whether criterion-related validity is used in a concurrent or predictive sense depends upon the intended use of the measuring instrument. If the intent is to assess the present status of individuals, then a concurrent approach is taken. If, however, the intent is to predict future behavior, then a predictive approach is needed.

When the approach is concurrent, the test and outside criterion are administered at the same time and the results of the two are correlated. For example, the concurrent validity of a newly constructed measure of anxiety might be assessed by comparing responses to it with responses to an already established measure of anxiety. If the resulting correlation is high, then concurrent validity can be supported.

When the approach is predictive, the outside criterion is not administered until a later date. If the correlation between the test and the outside criterion is high, the test in question is said to be predictive of the criterion. Predictive validity is frequently used in educational settings. For example, if one were interested in the predictive validity of grade point average in nursing courses for performance on state board examinations, the correlation between the two would supply the answer.

Construct Validity

A construct is composed of interrelated concepts. Because this sort of validity involves the measurement of abstractions, it is thought to be the most difficult. When a theoretical construct is formulated, construct validation procedures are used to decide whether the construct can be supported. Generally if scores on the instrument measuring the construct vary as predicted, construct validity is upheld. To speak of construct validity with confidence, a pattern of consistent findings involving different researchers should be established across time.

The basic steps in construct validation are shown in Table 8–7. Note that empirical relationships will not always be congruent with theoretical notions. When there is incongruence, researchers can consider one or more of the following. First, the instrument measuring the construct may be measuring something else. Second, it may be that the theoretical relationships are not correct. Third, it may be that the statistic or technique used to delineate the relationships was not appropriate.

Table 8–7. STEPS IN CONSTRUCT VALIDATION

1. The concepts or ideas involved in the construct are defined.
2. The relationships between the concepts or ideas are stated.
3. Measures of the concepts or ideas are formulated and administered.
4. The empirical relationships between the measures are identified.
5. The empirical relationships are interpreted in light of their clarification or support of the construct.

Construct validation techniques can be as simple as what is described as the known groups technique or as complex as the multitrait-multimethod approach described by Campbell and Fiske (1959). The underlying premise of the known groups technique is that groups inherently different are likely to differ on the trait or construct in question. For example, we might hypothesize that nurses or physicians who have been patients will be more empathetic than those who have not, as measured by an instrument designed to measure empathy. Following administration of the instrument, we would compare the two groups to determine if they differed significantly.

The multitrait-multimethod approach to construct validation is much more comprehensive. Several measures are used in this technique to determine convergence and discriminability. To document convergence different measures of the construct must produce similar results; that is, the measures should correlate highly with each other. Discriminability refers to ways in which the construct can be differentiated from other similar constructs. Here measures of similar but different constructs are administered and results should demonstrate differences.

EXAMPLES OF RELIABILITY AND VALIDITY

Cronbach's alpha; Test-Retest; Construct Validity. In a series of four studies, Dawson, Schirmer, and Beck (1984) demonstrated that their newly constructed Patient Self-Disclosure Instrument was internally consistent using Cronbach's alpha. They also demonstrated that the instrument was stable across time using test-related reliability procedures. Finally, they found that in separate tests of construct validity, patient self-disclosure was influenced by locus of control and perception of clinical empathy and that it covaried with heart rate changes.

Cronbach's alpha; Predictive (Criterion-Related) Validity. Miller and colleagues (1982) also used Cronbach's alpha to demonstrate the internal consistency of the Miller Attitude Scale designed to measure attitudes toward health. In addition, predictive validity of the scale was assessed by comparing patients' responses to the scale with responses to similar questions about the patients' health behavior obtained from a significant other or family member.

Construct Validity (Convergent and Discriminant Validity). In addition to using Cronbach's alpha to assess the internal consistency of their Patient Satisfaction Instrument, Hinshaw and Atwood (1982) assessed construct validity using the multitrait-multimethod approach. Validity estimates were obtained by noting the degree to which the traits measured by the Patient Satisfaction Instrument converged or diverged according to theoretical predictions.

ELEMENTS FOR CRITIQUE OF MEASUREMENT

- Are key variables quantified?
- Is the level of measurement described?
- Are there data to support the reliability of the measures?
- Are there data to support the validity of the measures?
- Is the level of precision of measurement consistent with the intent of the study?
- Are sources of measurement error acknowledged?

Questions and Activities

1. *How might the variable of "temperature" be operationalized at the nominal, ordinal, interval, and ratio levels?*
2. *What sources of error are controlled in the various approaches to reliability?*
3. *Discuss the notion that a test cannot be valid if it is not reliable.*
4. *Suppose you want to establish the validity of an instrument that measures pain. Describe the approaches you might take if you were assessing:*
   a. *Content validity*
   b. *Criterion-related validity*
   c. *Construct validity.*
5. *Describe how the level of measurement may dictate mathematical operations.*

Bibliography

Black, J. A., and Champion, D. J. (1976). *Methods and issues in social research.* New York: John Wiley and Sons.

Blalock, H. M. (1982). *Conceptualization and measurement in the social sciences.* Beverly Hills: Sage Publications.

Campbell, D. T., and Fiske, D. W. (1959). Convergent and discriminant validation by the multitrait-multimethod matrix. *Psychological Bulletin, 56*(2), 81–105.

Carmines, E. G., and Zeller, R. A. (1979). *Reliability and validity assessment.* Beverly Hills: Sage Publications.

Cronbach, L. J. (1951). Coefficient alpha and the internal structure of tests. *Psychometrika, 16*, 297–334.

Dawson, C., Schirmer, M., and Beck, L. (1984). A patient self-disclosure instrument. *Research in Nursing and Health, 7*(2), 135–147.

Dukes, W. F. (1965). N=1. *Psychological Bulletin, 64*, 74–79.

Ghiselli, E. E., Campbell, J. P., and Zedeck, S. (1981). *Measurement theory for the behavioral sciences.* San Francisco: W.H. Freeman.

Giovannetti, P. (1981). Aspects of measurement. In Y.M. Williamson (editor). *Research methodology and its application to nursing.* New York: John Wiley and Sons.

Gould, S. J. (1981). *The mismeasure of man.* New York: W.W. Norton.

Hinshaw, A. S., and Atwood, J. R. (1982). A patient satisfaction instrument: Precision by replication. *Nursing Research, 31*(3), 170–175.

Holm, K. (1983). Single subject research. *Nursing Research, 32*(4), 253–255.

Huck, S. W., Cormier, W. H., and Bounds, W. G., Jr. (1974). *Reading statistics and research.* New York: Harper and Row.

Kerlinger, F. N. (1973). *Foundations of behavioral research.* New York: Holt, Rinehart, and Winston.

Kuder, G. F., and Richardson, M. W. (1937). The theory of the estimation of test reliability. *Psychometrika, 2*, 151–160.

Miller, D. C. (1983). *Handbook of research design and social measurement.* 4th edition. New York: Longman.

Miller, P., Wikoff, R., McMahon, M., Garrett, M. J., and Johnson, N. (1982). Development of a health attitude scale. *Nursing Research, 31*(3), 132–136.

Plutchik, R. (1983). *Foundations of experimental research.* New York: Harper and Row.

Stevens, S. S. (1946). On the theory of scales of measurement. *Science, 103*(2684), 677–680.

Thorndike, R. L. (1982). *Applied psychometrics.* Boston: Houghton Mifflin.

Williamson, Y. M. (editor). (1981). *Research methodology and its application to nursing.* New York: John Wiley and Sons.

9

Sampling

OBJECTIVES

After completing this chapter the reader will be able to:

1. Differentiate between a population and a sample.
2. Discuss commonly used random and non-random sampling techniques.
3. Differentiate between randomization and random assignment.
4. Identify factors to consider in determining sample size.

It is not always feasible to collect data about everything or from everyone. Sampling makes it possible to arrive at general conclusions from studying a limited number of observations.

This chapter will begin with a discussion of the notions of population and sample fundamental to understanding the various approaches to sampling. As the chapter evolves, both probability and non-probability samples will be described.

POPULATIONS AND SAMPLES

A population can be defined as any large group of objects, people, or events that can be counted. Examples of populations include the institutionalized elderly, unwed teenaged mothers, or infants in the city of Chicago. Implicit in the notion of a population is the idea that, at least in principle, one can catalog or count every member even though it is not always reasonable to do so.

In research generalizations are made from a sample to a predefined population. Therefore a sample is merely a part of a population. Because a sample is used to describe a population, every attempt is made to select a sample that is representative. When attempting to clarify the ideas of population and sample it is important to realize that generalizations are made to a population using sample data. A population is thus the frame of reference. Generalizations cannot be made beyond a population as it is defined. Furthermore, a sample is always taken from a defined population.

Samples are not only useful but necessary. There are many situations where it is not practical or not possible to study all members of a population. For example, if one wished to make generalizations concerning health practices of middle-aged American women in the Washington, D.C., area, the most reasonable approach would be to select a sample from this defined population. Interestingly, data collected from such a sample may be better than data collected from every member of this population group. The reason is that there is less opportunity for error. A smaller number of people can be studied by a few highly trained personnel, whereas when attempts are made to study entire populations there is a greater risk of error. Inadequately trained research personnel, omitted or misrecorded information, and difficulties associated with handling and interpreting large volumes of data are but a few examples of errors that can occur.

SAMPLING METHODS

A sample should be chosen so a researcher is able as much as possible to see in the sample the characteristics of the population from which the sample was selected. It is an understatement to say that without careful attention to sampling, conclusions drawn from any study may be distorted and biased. The issue becomes one of how to select a sample so bias is kept at a minimum and generalizations can be readily made to a defined population.

As we shall see, statisticians advocate random sampling, that is, probability sampling, as the way to eliminate sampling bias. There are also other approaches to sampling that are not random but attempt to represent populations as closely as possible. Such approaches to sampling are called non-probability samples. Table 9–1 lists the approaches to sampling.

Probability Sample

With a probability sample each member of a population has an equal chance of being included in the sample. A probability sample is a random sample. When a random sample is obtained we assume that the sample is representative of the defined population, as all members of the population have an equal chance of being included.

Ideally the following conditions are required for probability samples (Table 9–2): First, the size of the population must be known. Second, the desired sample size must be specified. Finally, every element, person, or group must have an equal chance of being included in the sample. The most difficult conditions to satisfy are

Table 9–1. SUMMARY OF SAMPLING APPROACHES

1. Probability (random sample)	2. Non-probability
Simple random sample	Systematic sample
Stratified random sample	Convenience sample
Cluster sampling	Quota sample
Systematic sample	Accidental sample
	Purposive or judgmental sample
	Snowball sample
	3. Random assignment

Table 9–2. CONDITIONS FOR PROBABILITY SAMPLES

1. Size of the population known
2. Desired sample size specified
3. Every element or person has an equal chance of being included

the first and third. In regard to the first condition, many times it is not possible to know the exact size of a population. For example, to know the precise population of the city or state at any point in time is not a reasonable expectation, as the population is constantly in flux owing to births, deaths, and the migration of people. Because of this, the third condition, the expectation that every element or person has an equal chance of being included, is not totally realistic. The best any researcher can do in these situations is to use approximations of the totality of a population and randomly select a sample from the elements that are known.

Simple Random Sample. The most common type of probability sample is a simple random sample. The most rigorous approach to achieving this type of sample is to use a table of random numbers. In this method a number may be assigned to each member of a defined population. Those members are included in the sample whose numbers are taken from the table of random numbers.

A table of random numbers (an example of which appears in Table 9–3) can be entered in many ways. The usual approach is to

Table 9–3. AN EXAMPLE OF A TABLE OF RANDOM NUMBERS

64	20	64	31
75	19	40	19
16	12	37	80
72	92	84	68
65	04	23	02
43	30	37	10
33	98	42	98
76	18	62	94
66	96	63	39
35	01	33	15

enter at some arbitrary point, moving vertically down a column or columns of numbers until the desired sample is obtained. The number of columns used depends upon the sample size desired. Suppose that from a population of 900 people, a sample of 30 was desired. The table of random numbers is entered at an arbitrary point. Moving downward, the first 30 three-digit numbers (note that the first number in the adjacent column will be needed for use as the third digit) will be those selected to be part of the sample.

There are certain advantages to using a table of random numbers. The most important is that it is a good way to derive random samples from reasonably small populations. However, it is evident that such an approach would be tedious, as for example drawing a sample of 500 from a population of 25,000. But there is a solution to this dilemma, which is to use a computer program to generate a random sample from random numbers. This can be done with both large and small computers with relative ease. Another common method used to select a simple random sample is to write the names of an entire population on cards and randomly select a designated number.

Barsevick and Llewellyn (1982) used a modification of random sampling in a study of the effects of a towel bath on the anxiety level of patients anticipating invasive procedures and patients experiencing unrelieved pain. Patients who met criteria for the study were identified daily. A table of random numbers was used to determine which patients would be part of the study. The selection procedure was based on the assumption that patients available on any given day are representative of the target population. Patients were then randomly assigned to the towel bath or conventional bath groups.

Stratified Random Sample. When this approach is taken an investigator selects a sample absolutely representative of levels or parts of a significant factor or variable. For example, in a study of the influence of age on activity patterns, it would be very important to include individuals from many age groups. In this case the population could be divided into strata or groupings according to age and equal random samples drawn from each stratum.

A stratified random sample was used by Kirchhoff (1982) to secure a final sample of 240 accredited hospitals with critical care units. Hospitals were stratified according to bed size as follows: fewer than 100 beds, 100 to 199 beds, 200 to 299 beds, 300 to 399 beds, 400 to 499 beds, and more than 499 beds. Forty hospitals from each of the six strata were then randomly selected.

Cluster Sample. In cluster sampling, the population to be studied is divided into groups, and a random sample is then drawn from each group. Clusters are usually defined in terms of geographical location. If, for example, a survey of practicing American intensive care nurses was being attempted, a cluster sampling approach might be used. The initial step might be to divide the United States into geographic locations and obtain a list of hospitals in each location. The researcher would next randomly select specific hospitals in each region and then randomly select a given number of intensive care nurses from each.

Notice that cluster sampling involves more than one phase. In our example the first phase is the division of the country into regions, the second phase is obtaining a random sample of hospitals, and the third phase is randomly selecting nurses within each hospital. The group of hospitals selected in each region would constitute a cluster, and the nurses selected within each hospital would be a subgroup within the cluster.

Systematic Sample. Systematic sampling can also be used. Although not exactly random, it is convenient and practical. In systematic sampling members of the population are selected at a specific interval; for example, every other, or every third, fourth, or fifth member in a population may be taken into the sample. The trick here is that sampling begins with a random number.

Non-Probability Sample

A non-probability sample is one in which generalizations cannot be made to the population from which the sample was obtained. The reason is that all members or elements of the population do not have an equal chance of being included in the sample.

It would be unwise to think that non-probability samples are not useful. Many research situations do not require random samples, as for example in an exploratory study of a variable about which very little is known. This situation does not justify the additional time and expense required for a random sample. A non-probability sample can be obtained rapidly and with relative ease. Furthermore, there are ways to combine elements of randomness into a non-probability sample, as we shall see later.

Systematic Sample. This approach to sampling has already been discussed as a probability sampling method. It was said then and will be repeated now that systematic sampling is not entirely random. It includes elements of randomization, but the problem is that persons or elements between those selected are not considered for inclusion in the sample. Granted, the sampling procedure begins in a random way, but it is clear that selection of the remaining sample is not random. Therefore, because systematic sampling does not give every element in a population an equal chance of being included in the sample, generalizations about the population are limited.

Convenience Sample. A convenience sample is one in which all who agree to participate are taken into the study. A convenience sample uses people who happen to be available and are accessible to a researcher. For example, many psychological studies have been conducted by psychology professors who have used students as their samples. This is a convenient approach to sampling, as students are usually readily available to professors.

Longworth (1982) used a convenience sample consisting of 32 females recruited from the faculty, staff, and student population of a large Midwestern school of nursing to determine the psychophysiological effects of slow-stroke back massage in normotensive females. Slow-stroke back massage was perceived as relaxing by subjects as measured by an anxiety scale. Because the sample was a convenience sample, the researcher acknowledged that results could not be generalized to the general population.

Quota Sample. Convenience samples are not exactly the same as quota samples. When a quota sample is used, those who are available are selected to meet a certain quota, as for example a certain number of males and a certain number of females.

Accidental Sample. An accidental sample makes no attempt to include individuals or elements on the basis of certain criteria. Because anyone can be included in such a sample, it is economical of time and effort. Accidental samples may be used to pilot test a research protocol or questionnaire and because of this may prove very useful in the beginning phases of a study. The researcher should be aware, however, that it would not be wise to use an accidental sample when the intent is to come to a conclusion about a specific group of people or patients.

Purposive or Judgmental Sample. When an investigator attempts to ensure that specific elements are included in a sample, she is obtaining a judgmental or purposive sample, sometimes referred to as a quota sample. This approach employs a high degree of selectivity as the investigator is judging whether people have all of the necessary characteristics of the desired sample. An investigator uses judgmental or purposive sampling to guarantee that subjects will possess certain characteristics relevant to her research. Furthermore, an investigator can control the proportion of the desired sample characteristics so that the sample is as close as possible to a defined population.

Since such a sample is not random, the ability to generalize is limited, as with any non-probability sample. Furthermore, because judgmental or purposive samples are the non-random equivalent of stratified random samples, one might wonder why an investigator would go to such trouble to ensure that a sample represents certain characteristics of a population and not randomize. More than likely, practical considerations such as economy of time and effort are involved in the decision to use such an approach.

Some would argue that a purposive sample is inherently random. Here the reasoning is that an investigator really has no way of knowing who the people will be who will meet the sample criteria. For example, an investigator has little control over what people are hospitalized or are available in a clinic. This can be thought of as the clinical equivalent of randomization. But note that not all researchers will agree with this interpretation.

A two-stage sampling procedure was used to obtain subjects for a study of premenstrual muscle tension (Coyne, 1983). Initially 60 females responded to public notices advertising the study. They were given a symptom checklist and asked to rate on a scale from 0 to 10 the degree of discomfort they usually experienced premenstrually from 21 physiological and psychological symptoms. These scores were used to choose a sample of 24 women whose predicted premenstrual symptoms varied from no premenstrual distress to a high level of premenstrual distress.

Snowball Sample. The hallmark of a snowball sample is the use of initial members of a sample in the identification of others who might be appropriate participants in a study. Snowball samples have been used extensively in sociological studies where a specific behavior or characteristic seen in a few individuals is used to locate others who are similar. Because people tend to associate with others who are similar to themselves, on both a personal and professional basis, snowball sampling can be a very effective approach.

Random Assignment

When random sampling is employed, a population is first defined and a sample is randomly drawn from it. The idea is that because randomization is used, generalizations can be made back to the population. Often randomization in the strict sense is not possible. Many times sample criteria are delineated and an investigator, out of necessity, must include in the sample all those who meet sample criteria. Such occurrences are common in clinical research where persons meeting sample criteria are at a premium. How realistic is it then in such situations to use randomization?

First of all, do not forget that the idea of randomness is tied to the ability to make generalizations. When a sample is random, generalizations are readily made to a population. When a sample is not random, generalizations are not so easily made, but investigators can use random assignment to introduce randomness into a study. With random assignment, randomization procedures are used to place individuals into experimental or control groups. Random assignment comes after a sample has been obtained. Thus, in the situation where all individuals meeting sample criteria are included in a sample, randomization can still be used to assign subjects to groups. But when the results are obtained, generalizations can be made only to the sample actually observed.

Random assignment is also used following selection of a random sample. In such instances an investigator is guaranteeing two things. First of all, because the sample itself was randomly selected, generalizations can be made to a populaton. Second, the investigator is ensuring that any individual included in the sample has an equally likely chance of being included in any of the experimental treatment or control groups.

Flipping a coin is commonly used as a random assignment procedure. For example, when faced with the dilemma of deciding which patients who have met sampling criteria will be assigned to an experimental or control group, a flip of a coin can provide an objective approach. "Heads" can be used to signify the experimental group and "tails" the control group or vice versa. Because there is a 50/50 chance of heads or tails turning up with every flip of the coin, each subject has a 50/50 chance of being part of the experimental or control group.

SAMPLE SIZE

"How many subjects will I need in order to conduct my study?" is a question asked by every investigator. Often the decision is arbitrary or is a function of convention. It is usual for investigators to rely on an assumption of parametric statistics, namely a sample size of at least 30. A sample of at least 30 individuals supports the use of the more powerful statistical procedures, those that allow estimation of population values.

Many research texts advocate using as large a sample as possible. The primary rationale is that a large sample will be more likely to be representative of a population than a small sample. Note, however, that it is usually impossible to really know if a sample ever fully represents a population unless all of the characteristics of a population are known. On the other hand, if all of the characteristics of a population are known, a sample may not be needed. This has been referred to by many as the paradox of sampling.

There are ways to estimate sample size. One approach is the one-tenth rule suggesting that a sample should consist of one tenth of a population. Many times however a very credible investigation can be conducted using far less than one tenth of a population as a sample.

There are formulas that can be used to estimate sample size. To apply most formulas the level of significance, the amount of error the researcher is willing to tolerate, and an estimate of the sample standard deviation are needed. All three may be arbitrarily defined by an investigator.

Questions and Activities

1. *Differentiate between a sample and a population.*
2. *Discuss how you might obtain a random sample of nurses and/or students in your institution.*

ELEMENTS FOR CRITIQUE OF SAMPLING

- Does the researcher clearly describe the sampling procedure?
- Is the sample random or non-random?
- Are randomization procedures adequate?
- Does the researcher describe the representativeness of the sample to the population?
- Is the sample size adequate?
- Is there evidence of selection bias?
- If a non-random sample is used, is the distribution of key variables assessed?

3. *Why is a probability sample preferable to a non-probability sample?*
4. *What factors should be considered in a decision concerning sample size?*
5. *What is the difference between random assignment and random sampling?*

Bibliography

Barsevick, A., and Llewellyn, J. (1982). A comparison of the anxiety-reducing potential of two techniques of bathing. *Nursing Research, 31*(1), 22–27.

Coyne, C. (1983). Muscle tension and its relation to symptoms in the premenstruum. *Research in Nursing and Health, 6*(4), 199–206.

Kirchhoff, K. T. (1982). A diffusion survey of coronary precautions. *Nursing Research, 31*(4), 196–201.

Loevinger, J. (1965). Person and population as psychometric concepts. *Psychological Review, 72*, 143–155.

Longworth, J. C. D. (1982). Psychophysiological effects of slow stroke back massage in normotensive females. *Advances in Nursing Science, 4*(4), 44–61.

Sudman, S. (1982). *Applied sampling*. New York: Academic Press.

Williams, B. (1978). *A sampler on sampling*. New York: John Wiley and Sons.

IV

EVALUATING RESULTS

The objectives of this unit are to provide an overview of the various statistical techniques used by nurse researchers and to discuss key elements involved in data interpretation. Attention is given to both qualitative and quantitative analysis methods. Emphasis is placed not upon computation but upon the selection and application of specific statistical procedures.

10

Analysis of Data

OBJECTIVES

After completing this chapter the reader will be able to:

1. Describe the concept of hypothesis testing.
2. Discuss statistical concepts such as normal distribution, tests of significance, level of significance, and degrees of freedom.
3. Compare and contrast parametric and non-parametric methods.
4. Discuss commonly used descriptive statistics.
5. Describe commonly used inferential statistics.
6. List representative complex statistical procedures.
7. Identify specific correlational procedures.
8. Discuss approaches to qualitative data analysis.
9. Cite prevalent statistical problems.
10. Describe the role of the computer in data analysis.
11. Discuss the use of tables, graphs, and charts in data summary.

Florence Nightingale was a pioneer in solving problems with statistics. Upon return to England in July 1856, four months following the end of the Crimean War, she decided that the most appropriate recognition for her services would be to establish a commission to investigate military medical care (Cohen, 1984). She used statistics to convince people of the need for medical reform and consequently became a Fellow of the Royal Statistical Society and an honorary member of the American Statistical Association (Grier and Grier, 1978).

A statistic is a numerical value derived from sample data. Descriptive statistics describe, summarize, and characterize sample data, while inferential or parametric statistics are used to make projections or inferences to populations using sample data. There are two ways to make inferences or projections to populations: statistical estimation and hypothesis testing.

Statistical estimation is used to estimate a population value from sample data. For example, one can use the diastolic blood pressures obtained from a sample of hypertensives who have participated in a 12-week exercise program to estimate diastolic blood pressure from that population.

Table 10–1. EXAMPLE OF THE RELATION BETWEEN A RESEARCH AND A NULL HYPOTHESIS

Research Hypothesis	Null Hypothesis
Two groups differ according to blood pressure (Derived from theory)	Two groups have the same blood pressure (Based on research hypothesis)

Hypothesis Testing

As discussed in Chapter 3, a research hypothesis and a statistical hypothesis are not the same thing. A research hypothesis is an investigator's prediction of a specific outcome and is based upon theory. A statistical test is usually chosen to determine if the research hypothesis can be supported, but note that a statistical test does not directly test a research hypothesis. A statistical test evaluates a null hypothesis, often called a statistical hypothesis, to determine if statistical significance is present. A null hypothesis is stated in terms of no significant difference or relationship. Suppose a researcher predicts that exercises of the lower extremities such as walking or running will increase the bone content of the lumbar spine. The hypotheses would be as follows:

Null hypothesis: Lower extremity exercise will precipitate no significant change in the bone content of the lumbar spine.

Research hypothesis: Lower extremity exercise will precipitate increases in bone content of the lumbar spine.

Under the null hypothesis the researcher is expecting no change in bone as a consequence of exercise. Remember, however, that the researcher is hoping to reject the null hypothesis to support the research hypothesis. See Table 10–1 for an example of the relation

Figure 10–1. Normal distribution.

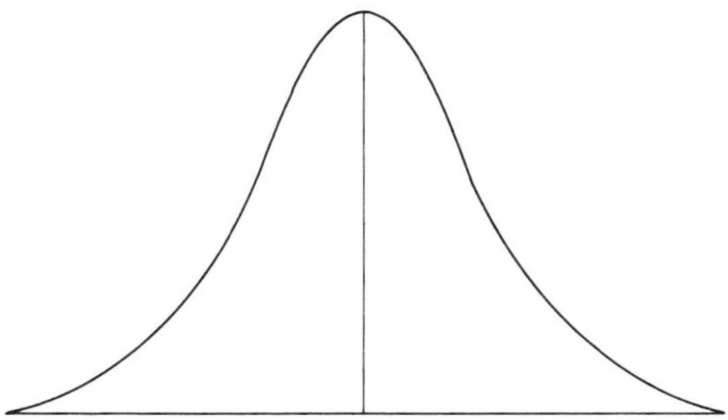

between a research hypothesis and a null hypothesis. Again it must be emphasized that a research hypothesis can never be proved but can only be supported, because actual population values are seldom known.

LANGUAGE OF STATISTICS

Normal Curve or Normal Distribution

The idea of a normal distribution represented by a bell-shaped curve (Figure 10–1) was first introduced by Gauss (1777–1855), a mathematician who observed that repeated measurements of the same phenomenon result in a regular sort of pattern. Specifically, the majority of observations tended to cluster around the mean, with an approximately equal number falling above and below the mean. Many human processes, such as heart rate, respiratory rate, or blood pressure, follow the pattern of a normal distribution. The concept of a normal distribution is an important one in statistics, as it is an assumption of many statistical tests.

One-Tailed or Two-Tailed Tests of Significance (Figure 10–2)

Every null hypothesis (H_0) has an alternate hypothesis (H_A) associated with it. The alternate hypothesis is actually the research hypothesis stated in symbolic terms. Suppose an investigator is studying an experimental group and a control group to determine the effectiveness of an experimental intervention. If she has no notion of the direction of the difference between the two groups, then a two-tailed statistical approach is warranted. This means that the alternate hypothesis is stated without claiming the direction of the difference between the experimental and control groups. The null hypothesis would look like this: H_0: $X_e = X_c$; the alternate hypothesis would look like this: H_A: $X_e \neq X_c$. Note that $\neq$ is the symbol for "not equal."

If the investigator did have an idea of the direction of the outcome, then a one-tailed statistical approach would be appropriate. This

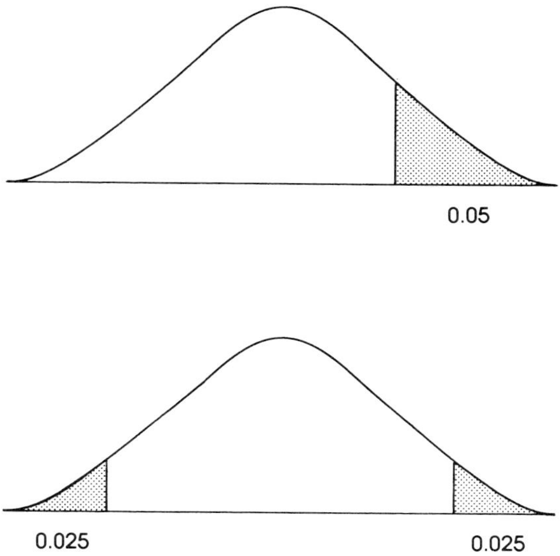

Figure 10–2. One-tailed and two-tailed tests.

means the investigator states that the experimental group is greater than (>) or less than (<) the control group. In this instance the null hypothesis would remain the same, but if the prediction were that the experimental group would exceed the control group, the alternate hypothesis would look like this: $H_A: X_e > X_c$.

Level of Significance

The level of significance, or alpha, is the probability of rejecting a null hypothesis when a null hypothesis is true. By convention 0.05 and 0.01 are the usual alpha levels that are chosen by investigators. If alpha is set at 0.05, an investigator can proclaim that she is 95 percent sure that rejecting the null hypothesis in support of the alternative hypothesis is correct. If alpha is set at 0.01 then an investigator is 99 percent sure.

Degrees of Freedom

The concept of degrees of freedom is of central importance in statistics. Simply stated, degrees of freedom are a measure of the number of independent observations in a data set. In the physical sciences the concept of degrees of freedom is used in reference to the movement of an object. An object that is free to move in one direction has one degree of freedom; an object that is free to move in two directions, two degrees of freedom; and three directions, three degrees of freedom.

Basically the same conceptual meaning is given to degrees of freedom in statistics. For any set of numbers, one number is always fixed and the rest are free to vary around the fixed number. To explain further, suppose that the sum of 25 numbers is a specific total. Only 24 of these numbers are independent, as one number must be the difference between the theoretically fixed total and the sum of the first 24 values. The degrees of freedom here is $N-1$ or $25-1 = 24$.

In order to use most statistical tables, one needs to know the degrees of freedom. Furthermore, many statistical tests incorporate degrees of freedom in their formulas.

Statistical Tables

Statistical tables are tables of probability values. The tables are entered at a specified alpha level and at particular degrees of freedom to locate a value termed the critical value. To cause a null hypothesis to be rejected, the calculated statistical value must exceed this critical value.

ASSUMPTIONS OF PARAMETRIC STATISTICS

Statistical assumptions are preconditions or requirements to be met before specific statistical tests are employed (Table 10–2). The assumptions of parametric statistics, the group of statistical tests using sample data to make inferences to specific populations, include

Table 10–2. ASSUMPTIONS OF PARAMETRIC STATISTICS

Normal distribution	Independence of observations
Random sampling	Interval scale measurement
Homogeneity of variance	Sample size greater than 30

normal distribution; random sampling; independence of observations; interval scale measurement; homogeneity of variance; and a sample of 30 or more observations, or $N > 30$.

Normal Distribution

Here it is implied that the values of the variable measured take the form of a normal or bell-shaped distribution. When a variable is normally distributed there are approximately equal numbers of observations falling above and below the mean or average score. It is said in statistical theory that as the number of observations increases, a sample distribution becomes increasingly normal. Again refer to Figure 10–1. Note that the greatest number of observations cluster around the mean. Note that when a distribution is normal the mean, median, and mode are identical.

Kurtosis refers to the "peakedness" of the curve (shown in Figure 10–3). When the normal curve is neither too tall and skinny nor too short and fat, it is labeled *mesokurtic*. A frequency distribution that is taller and skinnier than the normal distribution is called *leptokurtic*. A frequency distribution that is flatter, and more spread out, than a normal distribution is labeled *platykurtic*.

Random Sampling

To ensure as much as possible that a sample is representative of the population to which an investigator wishes to make inferences, random sampling should be used. There is error associated with any

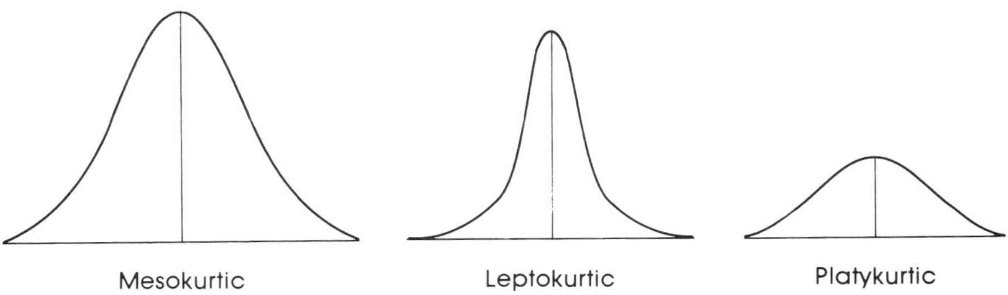

Figure 10–3. Examples of kurtosis.

sample, but random sampling theoretically supports the notion that error will be equally distributed.

When random sampling is used, the objective is to obtain unbiased sample values. Randomization may, however, be difficult to apply in a research setting. In many situations in nursing research randomization in the purest sense is not possible. Subjects included in a sample are those who are available and meet carefully delineated criteria. But modifications of randomization are better than no attempt to randomize. Selecting a sample by using a random start or randomly assigning subjects to treatment groups should be considered as a viable alternative to randomization.

Independence of Observations

If observations are not independent, the laws of chance do not operate. Therefore, this assumption is a relatively important one. When observations are independent the occurrence of one score or value in no way influences the occurrence of other scores on subsequent trials. Suppose that an experiment necessitated that repeated measurements be made of blood pressure. To ensure independence of observations the investigator would have to allow sufficient time between measurements so that a previous blood pressure reading would not influence the next blood pressure.

Interval Scale Measurement

With measurements that are interval scale or approximately interval scale (such as many psychological and behavioral measures), mathematical operations associated with parametric statistical tests can be readily applied. Remember that observations made using an interval measurement scale can be ordered and that the distance between each and every pair of observations can be quantitatively measured.

Additivity is an underlying assumption of the interval scale. Theoretically the distance between observed points can be added together. For example, if three people were standing in line, the distance between person 1 and person 2 plus the distance between

Table 10–3. FOUR SCALES OF MEASUREMENT AND APPROPRIATE STATISTICS

Scale of Measurement	Statistics
Nominal	Chi-square
Ordinal	Rank-order statistics
Interval	t-Test, analysis of variance, correlation
Ratio	t-Test, analysis of variance, correlation

person 2 and person 3 can be added to get the distance between person 1 and person 3. This notion of additivity is easily verified with physical measurement, but it must be realized that it is not quite so easy with behavioral measurements. Table 10–3 lists each level of measurement, along with statistics commonly associated with each.

It should be noted that many question whether a distinction between ordinal and interval level measurement should be made. Many researchers prefer to use parametric statistics even when data are ordinal, as they are more apt to detect significant differences when significant differences are present. In other words, parametric tests are more powerful.

ASSUMPTIONS OF NON-PARAMETRIC STATISTICS

Non-parametric statistical tests are not bound by the many assumptions of parametric tests. Generally, non-parameteric tests are free of assumptions about the characteristics of the sampling distribution and do not assume that data are at the interval level of measurement. Furthermore, non-parametric tests are designed for small samples, specifically those less than 30. However, non-parametric tests are less powerful.

STATISTICAL PROCEDURES

This section will be devoted to (1) descriptive statistics; (2) commonly used inferential statistics; and (3) complex statistics.

Descriptive Statistics

Descriptive statistics are summary statistics, useful for describing a set of numbers. Most often these numbers are obtained from a particular sample or group. Descriptive statistics describe collective characteristics of a given body of data and, more important, help in looking at sample data in real-world terms.

Included in this branch of statistics are particularly useful procedures for organizing, summarizing, and interpreting data. No matter what other statistical procedures are to be used, data obtained from any research study should initially be presented using descriptive statistical methods.

The most common descriptive statistical procedures are listed in Table 10–4. As will be demonstrated, each provides different information about a set of numbers. It should be noted that many research papers neglect to provide the reader with descriptive statistical information. As we shall see, valuable information is being lost that in many situations may help the reader to better interpret results.

Measures of Central Tendency

The mode, median, and mean are the most frequently used measures of central tendency. Of the three, the mode is the least complex and is defined as the observation or number that occurs the greatest number of times. In the distribution of numbers shown in Example 1 in Table 10–5, the mode is 3, as it is the most frequently occurring number.

Identifying the mode is not always so simple. Sometimes a distribution of numbers has more than one mode. In this instance all should be identified. Looking at the numbers in Example 2 in Table 10–5, it is clear that there are two modes, thus rendering this distribution of numbers bimodal.

Table 10–4. COMMON DESCRIPTIVE STATISTICS

Frequency distributions	Measures of dispersion
Measures of central tendency	Range
Mean	Variance
Mode	Standard deviation
Median	

Table 10–5. DERIVING MEASURES OF CENTRAL TENDENCY: THE MODE

Example 1:	2, 3, 3, 5, 6, 7, 9
Example 2:	2, 3, 3, 5, 6, 6, 7, 9
Example 3:	2, 2, 3, 3, 5, 5, 6, 6, 7, 7, 9, 9

The mode is useful in describing a distribution of numbers only when a few observations occur with greater frequency than all others. It is not very useful, however, when numbers occur with equal frequency, as shown in Example 3 in Table 10–5. It is clear that it is impossible here to describe the most frequently occurring number.

Another commonly used measure of central tendency is the median or midpoint of a group of observations. To derive the median, it is usual to arrange numbers in order of magnitude and subsequently identify the point at which 50 percent of the observations are above and 50 percent are below. Look now at Example 1 in Table 10–6. The median of this group of numbers is 5, as it is at this point that this distribution of numbers is divided in half.

There is at least one additional situation in which finding the median is a bit more difficult. It occurs when a distribution contains an even number of observations. As seen in Example 2 in Table 10–6, where there are 10 observations, the median is not easily identified. To find the median here, the middle two numbers (i.e., 5 and 6) are averaged as shown in Example 3 in Table 10–6.

The mean is the arithmetic average of a group of numbers. It is found by summing a group of observations and dividing by the number of observations. Example 1 in Table 10–7 presents the statistical formula for deriving the mean. Note that the symbol is the Greek capital letter sigma (Σ). It is used in statistics to indicate that numbers are to be added together or summed. The X following is used to signify a particular variable whose values are to be added

Table 10–6. DERIVING MEASURES OF CENTRAL TENDENCY: THE MEDIAN

Example 1:	1, 2, 3, 4, 5, 6, 7, 8, 9
Example 2:	1, 2, 3, 4, 5, 6, 7, 8, 9, 10
Example 3:	$\frac{5 + 6}{2} = 5.5$

Table 10–7. DERIVING THE MEAN

$$\text{Example 1: } {}^{*}\,\overline{X} = \frac{\Sigma X}{N}$$

$$\text{Example 2: } {}^{*}\,\overline{X} = \frac{x_1 + x_2 + x_3 \ldots x_n}{N}$$

*When N is equal to the total number of observations.

together. Realize here that the values of X are signified by a lower case or small x, while the upper case or capital X is really composed of many small x's, as shown in Example 2 in Table 10–7.

Looking again to the formula for the arithmetic mean, it should be pointed out that $\bar{X}$ is the conventional symbol for the mean. Many other statistical formulas use $\bar{X}$, so you will be exposed to this symbol again. The mean is very sensitive to extreme scores and as a consequence has the tendency to be pulled toward the extreme. For instance, one millionaire in a group of ten people can cause the average income to be much higher than it would be without the millionaire. The examples given in Table 10–8 illustrate this phenomenon. Whether one is a consumer or practitioner of research, one must realize that the mean is derived by an averaging process and can be strongly influenced by a limited number of extreme values. When this occurs, potentially important information from a few individuals may be ignored.

Measures of Dispersion

Measures of dispersion include the range, the standard deviation, and the variance. Each of these statistics provides a measure of the amount of variation in a group of observations. If we considered an individ-

Table 10–8. EXTREME SCORES AND THE MEAN

$$\text{Example 1: } \frac{2 + 3 + 3 + 5 + 6 + 7 + 9}{7} = 5$$

$$\text{Example 2: } \frac{2 + 3 + 3 + 5 + 6 + 30 + 16}{7} = 9.3$$

$$\text{Example 3: } \frac{1 + 1 + 1 + 5 + 5 + 6 + 6}{7} = 3.6$$

Table 10–9. THE RANGE

Range = H − L
Where H = highest value
L = lowest value
Example: Given the following set of observations, derive the range
2.5, 10, 25, 52
Range = H − L
= 52 − 2.5 = 49.5

ual's weight on a day-by-day basis, we would see that it would fluctuate or vary.

The range is the least complex measure and provides at best a crude indicator. To derive the range the lowest value in a set of numbers is subtracted from the highest value. Table 10–9 presents the standard formula for the range and an example of how it is applied.

Although the range provides one indicator of how scores or numbers in a distribution vary, it is at best a crude way to describe the dispersion of a set of numbers. The reason is that the range is dependent upon extreme scores. Look at the simple formula for the range, H − L. Keeping all values constant except the highest value, the range can change drastically. The range of 2, 3, 4, 5, 6, 50 is 48. It may be that 50 is a spurious value; when only the range of this data set is presented or discussed, one can easily be misled.

The variance and standard deviation are more complex mathematically but provide more information than the range. The variance is defined as the average of squared deviations from the mean, while the standard deviation is the square root of the variance. There is a distinction between the population's and the sample's standard deviation and variance. Refer now to Table 10–10. The Greek symbol σ is used to denote population parameters, while the letter S is used when the focus is the sample variance and standard deviation. Most often the population values are not known and therefore you will rely on sample values.

Table 10–10. VARIANCE AND STANDARD DEVIATION

	Population	**Sample**
Variance	σ^2	S^2
Standard deviation	σ	S

Table 10–11. FREQUENCY DISTRIBUTION OF DIASTOLIC BLOOD PRESSURE (DBP) FOR A SAMPLE OF MIDDLE-AGED ATHLETES (N = 29)

DBP	Frequency
74	6
73	5
70	5
69	4
68	2
67	2
65	2
63	2
62	1

Frequency Distributions

A frequency distribution summarizes raw data. The simplest form it takes is illustrated by Table 10–11. Although the frequency of each diastolic pressure value does not vary to any great extent, it is apparent that more individuals in this sample have higher diastolic pressures. From looking at this display of values one can get an idea as to the shape the distribution would take if diastolic values were plotted on a graph.

There are other approaches to constructing a frequency distribution. One combines scores into groups and displays the frequency of scores falling into the respective score groupings. The primary advantage here is that the number of lines on the frequency table is decreased, since each individual score is not displayed. Table 10–12 gives an example of a grouped frequency distribution. Note how much simpler the distribution appears as it functions to summarize the

Table 10–12. GROUPED FREQUENCY DISTRIBUTION OF BODY WEIGHT IN POUNDS OF A SAMPLE OF FEMALE RUNNERS (N = 27)

Grouped Values	Frequency
105–110	8
100–104	8
95–99	6
90–94	5

Table 10–13. CUMULATIVE FREQUENCY OF PHYSIOLOGY TEST SCORES FOR A CLASS OF FIRST-YEAR GRADUATE STUDENTS

Score Range	Frequency	Cumulative Frequency	Cumulative Percent
80–84	1	40	100
75–79	2	39	97.5
70–74	4	37	92.5
65–69	3	33	82.5
60–64	6	30	75
55–59	5	24	60
50–54	3	19	47.5
45–49	5	16	40
40–44	3	11	27.5
35–39	5	8	20
30–34	1	3	7.5
25–29	2	2	5

frequency with which each score or value falls within a certain interval rather than listing every score.

Another kind of frequency distribution is the cumulative frequency distribution as shown in Table 10–13. The first two columns are a grouped frequency distribution. The third column is what makes a cumulative frequency distribution unique. This column demonstrates a running total beginning at the lowest score range. The total number of students in the physiology class is 40. Two students received a grade falling in the 25–29 range, while in the next class interval one student scored in the 30–40 range. It can be seen that this student added one to the cumulative frequency.

Commonly Used Inferential Statistical Procedures

Now the commonly used statistical procedures will be described. Inferential statistics are used to test hypotheses. In many instances reference will be made to the steps involved in hypothesis testing shown in Table 10–14. It should be noted that statistical tests have unique null hypotheses. This will be more understandable as we learn the kind of information each test was designed to supply.

Table 10–14. STEPS IN HYPOTHESIS TESTING

1. State the null or statistical hypothesis (H_0).
   Then state the alternate hypothesis (H_A).
2. Choose the level of significance.
3. Choose the statistic.
4. Find the critical statistical value from the appropriate statistical table.
5. Define the rejection rule.
6. Calculate the statistic.
7. Reject or do not reject the null hypothesis.

The t-Test

The t-test is a parametric statistic that is widely used in research. There are three kinds of t-tests. The first, known as the one-sample t-test, is used to test the null hypothesis that a mean is equal to a specific value. The second is a two-sample t-test used to test the null hypothesis that the means of two groups are equal to each other. The third, the correlated t-test, is used to determine if a particular group's scores on two variables are significantly different.

Consider a situation in which an investigator is interested in the effect of a disease state on serum potassium level. If the mean serum potassium of the population to which the investigator wishes to make inferences is known to be 4.5 and the mean of the sample ($N = 10$) exhibiting the disease is 3.4, then a one-sample t-test is the appropriate statistic.

To test whether the sample mean is significantly different from the population mean, the investigator would proceed as shown in Table 10–15.

A t-test may also be used to test the difference between two means. Table 10–16 illustrates such a situation. Depicted are scores on leadership of two groups of staff nurses: the first group attended a two-week seminar in leadership (experimental group), while the second group did not (control group). Using the t-test to evaluate whether the two groups differed significantly in terms of leadership, the investigator subjected the data to a t-test (Table 10–17). Notice that this formula is different from the formula in Table 10–15 in two ways. First, the numerator assesses the absolute difference between the sample and population means. Second, in the denominator is the formula for the pooled variance, which is used when the population variance is not known. To obtain the pooled variance, the squared

Table 10–15. TESTING A HYPOTHESIS WITH A ONE-SAMPLE t-TEST

1. Null hypothesis (H_0): X = 4.5
   Alternate (H_A): X ≠ 4.5
2. Level of significance = 0.01
3. Statistic = t-test
   Formula: $t = \frac{\overline{X} - \mu}{S/\sqrt{n}}$
   Where $\overline{X}$ = sample mean
   μ = population mean
   s = sample standard deviation
4. Define rejection region
   Degrees of freedom = n − 1 = 9
   Level of significance is divided in half because there is not a direction specified in H_A
   The t table it is entered at 9 degrees of freedom and the 0.005 level of significance. The critical value is 3.25.
5. Rejection rule: Reject H_0 if t < or > 3.25
6. $t = \frac{3.4 - 4.5}{0.16} = -6.9$
7. Reject H_0

deviations from the means of the two samples are pooled to provide an estimate of the population variance.

Chi-Square

The chi-square statistic (Table 10–18) tests the independence of variables by measuring the discrepancy between observed and expected frequencies. It is a non-parametric statistic. The general formula for chi-square as well as an example is shown in Table 10–18. The chi-square distribution has different shapes and values depending upon the degrees of freedom. The degrees of freedom can be computed

Table 10–16. LEADERSHIP SCORES

Experimental (N=5)	Control (N=5)
60.2	61.3
61.3	60.0
57.5	59.8
58.9	59.1
62.0	63.0

Table 10–17. t-TEST FOR SAMPLE MEANS

1. $H_0: X_E - X_c = 0$
   $H_A: X_E - X_c = 0$
2. Level of significance = 0.05
3. $t = \dfrac{(X_E - X_c)}{Sp\sqrt{1/n_e + 1/n_c}}$

   $$\text{Where } Sp = \sqrt{\frac{(n_E - 1)\,S_E^2 + (n_c - 1)S_c^2}{n_E + n_c - 2}}$$

4. Critical value at:
   $df = n_E + n_c - 2 = 8$
   $\alpha\ 0.05/2 = 0.025$
   $= 2.3060$
5. Reject H_0 if $t > 2.3060$ or < -2.3060
6. $t = -0.620$
7. Do not reject H_0

by: df = $(r-1) \times (c-1)$; r = number of rows in the table; c = number of columns.

Look at Table 10–18, part 2. The boxes, called cells, and the numbers outside the boxes, called marginal totals, compose the contingency table. If the number of observations is less than 20, or if any one of the cells in the contingency table has fewer than 5 observations, we cannot use the chi-square formula and must use the Fisher exact probability test.

Table 10–18. CHI SQUARE

1. $X^2 = \dfrac{(O - E)^2}{E}$ Where O = Observed frequencies, E = Expected frequencies

2. Stress

Sex	High	Low	
Male	12	4	16
Female	8	8	16
	20	12	32

3. $C = \dfrac{X^2}{X^2 + N}$

The *contingency coefficient* (C) (Table 10–18, part 3) can be calculated following a chi-square to express the degree of relatedness between two nominal variables. The larger the value of C, the greater the degree of relatedness.

Analysis of Variance (ANOVA)

Analysis of variance, known as the F ratio, is used for determining whether two or more group variances differ from one another to a significant extent or merely by chance. It is a parametric statistic. The answer provided by the F ratio is whether a statistically significant variation exists among group means. The null or statistical hypothesis is that the groups are equal. In other words, Group 1 = Group 2 = Group 3. If the groups are not equal, the resulting F ratio will be greater than 1. The logic of analysis of variance becomes clear when the components of the formula are considered.

$$F = \frac{\text{Variance between groups}}{\text{Variance within groups}}$$

The numerator of the formula is the information that an investigator is seeking—that is, do the groups involved in an experiment differ from one another? One of the groups may be a control group and the others experimental groups. The denominator of the formula is the error component. When groups are homogeneous, the error is small and the resulting F ratio will have a tendency to be larger. When groups are not homogeneous, the difference within groups may be greater than the difference between groups and the resulting F ratio will be small and possibly insignificant. For purposes of illustration, suppose the variance between groups is 10 and the variance within groups is 2 (relatively small error); then the resulting F ratio would be 5. If, however, the variance within groups increased to 7 (relatively large error), the resulting F ratio (10/7) would be much smaller, specifically 1.43. It should be noted that when the resulting F ratio is statistically significant, another group of statistical tests known as post hoc comparison tests are used to locate the specific source of the significance. Holm and Christman (1985) define each of these tests and give guidelines for their application.

Complex Statistics

In this section the most commonly used complex statistics are summarized. The intent is to give you a basic idea of how these procedures are used so you can begin to read research reports using these procedures. At best we offer but a brief overview. If you have further questions or wish a more complete understanding, consult with a statistician or researcher or refer to a more detailed research text.

Analysis of Covariance

There are two ways to reduce error in an experiment. One is to use experimental or direct control, such as increasing the uniformity of conditions under which the experiment is run or increasing the accuracy of the measurement. The second way is to use statistical control, also referred to as the analysis of covariance. This enables an investigator to increase the precision of an experiment by removing potential sources of bias that are difficult to eliminate by experimental control. Analysis of covariance combines the basic ideas of analysis of variance and correlational analysis.

A covariate (also called a concomitant variate) is a source of variation that cannot be controlled in an experiment. A covariate may influence measurement of a dependent variable. For example, in a study designed to test the results of four programs to increase the mathematical ability of four groups of nursing students, we might measure the mathematical ability of each student at the end of the programs. Because we cannot directly control the differences in mathematical ability before the students are exposed to a program, it would be wise to use analysis of covariance. This procedure will make adjustments in the dependent variable, specifically the score on mathematical ability at the end of the programs, for initial differences in mathematical ability between the groups. This will enable us to isolate the effects of the four programs and determine which offers the best results.

Multiple Regression

Multiple regression is a procedure used to view the relationship between a dependent variable and a set of independent or predictor variables. For example, an investigator might be interested in determining how grades in the basic sciences influenced state board scores in medical-surgical nursing. The dependent variable in this case is the state board scores, while grades in basic science courses are the independent variables.

Discriminant Function Analysis

Discriminant function analysis answers the question: How can individuals best be assigned to groups on the basis of several variables? This procedure is similar to multiple regression, except that the dependent variable, instead of being a score, is a group or category. Discriminant function might be used to build a physical and psychological profile of the individual most likely to continue with an exercise program.

Canonical Correlation

Canonical correlation is another complex statistical procedure. It is appropriate for correlating many independent variables with many dependent variables. This procedure might be used to correlate personality variables with job satisfaction variables.

Factor Analysis

Factor analysis is a data-reduction technique useful for determining if variables share something in common. It is useful for explaining relationships among many variables in a simplified way. Factor analysis is often used to support the validity of a measuring instrument. Jalowiec, Murphy, and Powers (1984) factor analyzed 40 coping behaviors to determine if a previously established classification of coping behavior (problem-oriented vs. affective-oriented) was valid. They found the variables that were predominantly problem-oriented coping strategies were highly related with each other and clustered together (factor 1), and variables clustering on the second factor were primarily affective-oriented (factor 2). These researchers were thus able to validate what had previously been determined by 20 nurse judges using factor analysis.

Table 10–19. ROUGH GUIDE TO INTERPRETING CORRELATIONS

< 0.30, low	0.70 to 0.90, high
0.30 to 0.70, moderate	> 0.90, very high

CORRELATIONAL STATISTICS

There are a number of statistics used to examine the relationships between variables. It is wise to be familiar with the most commonly used correlational statistics.

Pearson product-moment correlation (r) is used to measure the relationship between two continuous variables. The stability of this correlation increases as the number of observations increases. A Pearson correlation is stable when it is statistically significant. It is important to realize that even a low correlation can be stable, that is, statistically significant, if the number of observations is large. Strength or magnitude of a correlation is another matter. Table 10–19 presents a rough guide to interpreting the magnitude of a correlation.

Multiple correlation (R) is a procedure used to examine the relationships between at least three variables.

Phi coefficient measures the degree of relationship between two nominal dichotomous variables.

Point biserial correlation assesses the relationship between one continuous and one truly dichotomous variable.

Biserial correlation measures the relationship between a continuous variable and one that is forced into a dichotomy.

Partial correlation is used to measure the relationship of two continuous variables, controlling for the effects of a third variable by holding it constant.

Eta is for measuring the relationship between two continuous curvilinear variables.

Spearman's rho measures the relationship between two ordinal variables. *Gamma* is a similar statistic.

NON–PARAMETRIC STATISTICS

As mentioned earlier, non-parametric statistics are not based on assumptions about a sample's parent population. Non-parametric

Table 10–20. NON-PARAMETRIC STATISTICS

	One-Sample	Two-Sample Unrelated	Two-Sample Related
Nominal	Binominal Chi-square	Fisher exact test Chi-square	McNemar test
Ordinal	Kolmogorov-Smirnov one-sample One-sample runs test	Median test Kolmogorov-Smirnov two-sample	Sign test Wilcoxin Mann-Whitney U
Interval	—	—	Walsh test Randomization test

statistics are used when a researcher does not wish to violate parametric assumptions. Be aware, however, that non-parametric tests, while relatively easy to use, are less powerful, that is, less apt to detect significant differences when differences are present.

Table 10–20 is a guide to commonly used non-parametric statistics taken from Siegel's (1956) classic text on the subject. The table is not all-inconclusive, as Siegel describes at least ten times as many tests.

Table 10–21 presents another useful chart. Listed here are the non-parametric counterparts of commonly used parametric statistics.

ANALYSIS OF QUALITATIVE DATA

The statistical procedures we have discussed thus far are based on research methods that emphasize measurable findings, that is, findings to which a number can be easily attached. Analysis of qualitative

Table 10–21. NON-PARAMETRIC COUNTERPARTS OF COMMON PARAMETRIC TESTS

Non-Parametric	Parametric
1. Spearman's rho	1. Pearson r
2. Mann-Whitney U	2. t-Test
3. Kruskall-Wallis	3. One-way analysis of variance
4. Friedman	4. Two-way analysis of variance

data is not quite that simple. Qualitative methods focus on, for instance, such things as beliefs, meanings, attributes, and symbols, all of which are difficult to quantify. Qualitative data are often obtained by observational methods or by interviewers using open-ended questions that are impossible to translate directly into numbers.

Qualitative researchers often use content analysis procedures to analyze their data. Content analysis is a technique used to make replicable and valid inferences from qualitative data. Content analysis can be done at a manifest level, meaning that what is said or what is observed is coded directly, or at a latent level, where the perceived meaning of the response or perceptions of the underlying dynamics of the response are coded.

An excellent example of content analysis is given by Powers, Murphy, and Wooldridge (1983). From a total pool of 88 typed transcripts of nurse-patient interactions in a hypertension education program, 62 were chosen on the basis of completeness of content. Following a thorough review of the transcripts and the teaching checklist used as a content guide by the nurses, a pilot categorization scheme was constructed. Initially 32 categories were identified based upon the teaching checklist, including concept of blood pressure, measurement of blood pressure and blood pressure values, concept of hypertension as a lifelong disease, risk factors and complications, basic pathology of hypertension, rationale for treatment, medication schedules and side effects, dietary restrictions, weight control and exercise, smoking, and stress/lifestyle. Each verbal exchange between a nurse and patient provided the unit of analysis. A verbal exchange was defined as one complete statement by a nurse followed by a patient response. The investigators had now created a framework for analyzing each of the typed transcripts.

PREVALENT STATISTICAL PROBLEMS

From a review of the contemporary nursing research literature Reid (1983) noted three prevalent statistical problems (Table 10–22) centering on lack of protection against Type I error, which is falsely rejecting a null hypothesis (see Table 11–2). The first, using a t-test to compare more than a single set of means, increases the level of significance (alpha). When, for example, alpha is set at 0.05 and three

Table 10–22. STATISTICAL APPROACHES LEADING TO TYPE I ERROR*

Initial use of the t-test to compare more than one set of means
Use of the t-test to compare Pearson correlation coefficients
Not using a multivariate statistic

*Copyright 1983, American Journal of Nursing Company. Reprinted with permission from Reid, B. J.: Potential sources of type I error and possible solutions to avoid a "galloping" alpha rate. *Nursing Research, 32*(3): 190–191, 1983.

independent t-tests are performed, alpha really is not 0.05 but 0.1427. This is calculated as follows:

$$1-[(1-0.05)^3]=$$
$$1-0.8573 \text{ or } 0.1427$$

It is clear that the probability of falsely rejecting the null hypothesis has escalated. Such may occur in a study using more than two groups. When assessing the impact of children's locus of control beliefs on preoperative coping behavior, Lamotagne (1984) divided children into three groups: active copers; avoidant copers; and combination active-avoidant. Analysis of variance was used to determine if the three groups differed significantly on locus of control scores. Statistical significance was achieved at < 0.05. This researcher did not fall victim to using t-tests to compare the differences but chose analysis of variance, the correct procedure. Unlike the t-test, analysis of variance is designed for use with two or more groups. Multiple t-tests violate the assumption of two randomly drawn independent samples.

The next two situations cited by Reid—using t-tests to compare two correlation coefficients or using a univariate statistic when a multivariate statistic is more appropriate—are both questionable practices. The level of alpha inflates and the risk of falsely rejecting a null hypothesis increases.

USING THE COMPUTER FOR DATA ANALYSIS

The computer has had a tremendous impact on data analysis. It is no longer necessary for researchers to perform manually the tedious calculations associated with many statistical procedures and large sample sizes. Computers not only are less prone to computational error but perform calculations far faster than humans. Because of computers, researchers can spend more time interpreting data.

There are many statistical programs available for both large and small computers. Only when browsing through the software program catalogs available in most bookstores can one fully appreciate the number of statistical programs available for the small computer. The larger mainframe computers located at most universities and medical centers can use more comprehensive statistical programs such as SPSS (Statistical Package for the Social Sciences) and SAS (Statistical Analysis System). Each has the capability of performing most statistical calculations.

TABLES, GRAPHS, AND CHARTS

Statistics are used to answer research questions. When planning an analysis it is wise to allow time to become familiar with the data. First, descriptive statistics should be computed for all key variables. Second, data might be displayed in charts and graphs to increase the researcher's familiarity. Tabular and graphic presentations of data are often preferable, because they can make it easier to visualize key relationships. Although these visual representations are sometimes difficult to construct and represent added expense in terms of typing and publication, they can actually be economical because they can serve to compress lengthy text and make it more relevant. The *Publication Manual of the American Psychological Association* clearly summarizes the key points in constructing tables and graphs and is recommended for further reference.

Tables

A table displays data in rows and columns. While the essential ingredients of a table are highlighted in the text, a good table should stand alone. The text should never repeat information more easily derived from a table; such redundancy is needless. In the same light, a table should be able to stand alone without the text to explain it.

Tables should always be designed with the convenience of the reader foremost in mind. They should always be placed at a convenient point within the text, so that the reader does not have to turn to the next page or turn the document sideways to read it.

Parts of a Table

The parts of a table are illustrated in Table 10–23.

1. Title. Each table must have a brief but clearly explanatory title. The title is always accompanied by a number that is referenced in the text.

2. Columns. Arrangements of vertical data.

Table 10–23. ILLUSTRATION OF PARTS OF A TABLE

(1) **Table 8. Mean Scores on Knowledge Tests of Cardiovascular Surgery Patients with and without Structured Teaching**

(5b) *Group*	*n*[a]	*Preop*	*Postop*
Coronary artery bypass patients			
Structured teaching	20 (18)	280	319
Unstructured teaching	20 (19)	240	263
Peripheral vascular patients			
Structured teaching	20 (19)	281	317
Unstructured teaching	20 (20)	232	262

(7a) *Note*. Maximum score = 320.

(7b) [a]Numbers in parentheses indicate the number of patients who completed both tests.

3. Rows. Arrangements of horizontal data.

4. Cells. Small spaces defined by the intersection of a column and a row.

5. Column Headings. The left hand column is composed of the headings of the rows and is called the *stub* (5a). This column has a heading called a *stubhead* (5b). The other vertical columns are identified with *boxheads* (5c). If a boxhead extends over more than one column, it is called a *subheading*.

6. Body. All the cells in a table.

7. Notes. Used to further explain abbreviations, italics, parentheses, and units of measurement. Notes can be general (7a) (relating to the table as a whole) or specific (7b) (referring to a particular column or individual entry).

Graphs

A graph (also referred to as a figure or diagram) is a visual representation of the data that allows the reader to get an overall impression of the shape of a score distribution, or to get a quick idea of how several groups compare. Like tables, graphs are used to increase the reader's understanding of the text. Figures and graphs are even more expensive than tables, so the writer should always ask:

1. Will it enhance or clarify the text?
2. Is it necessary or only repetitious?

Figures and graphs should be of professional quality, never hand-drawn. It is possible for a researcher to use press-on letters or other commercially available aids to create an attractive graph. Computer-generated figures are increasing in popularity and are an acceptable alternative.

Parts of a Graph

The parts of a graph are shown in Figure 10–4.

1. Title. Like a table, a graph, figure, or diagram should be clearly and concisely labeled with a number referenced in the text.

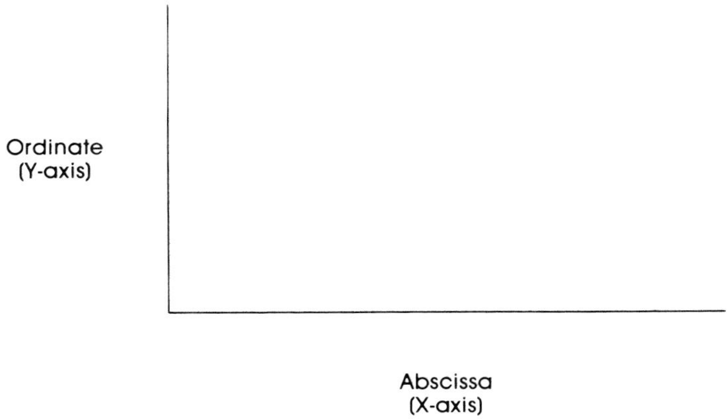

Figure 10–4. Parts of a graph.

2. **Abscissa.** The horizontal scale of a graph, also called the "x-axis."
3. **Ordinate.** The vertical scale of a graph, also called the "y-axis."

Types of Graphs

Pie Chart. A pie chart (shown in Figure 10–5) is a circle in which the 360 degrees are used to represent 100 percent of the sample. Pie

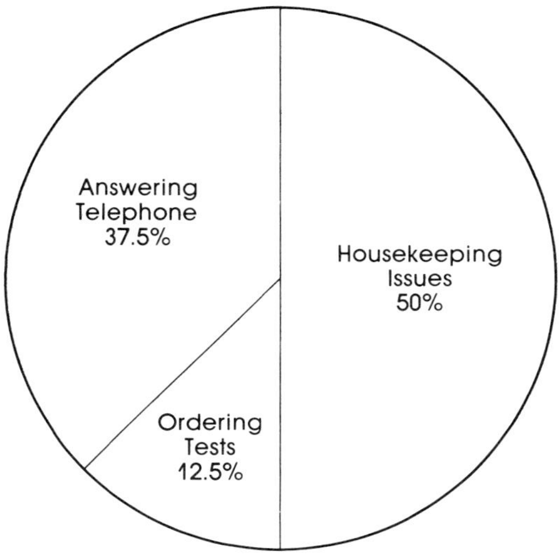

Figure 10–5. Pie chart. Diagram represents the distribution of non-nursing time spent on various tasks by the average staff nurse. (Fictitious data.)

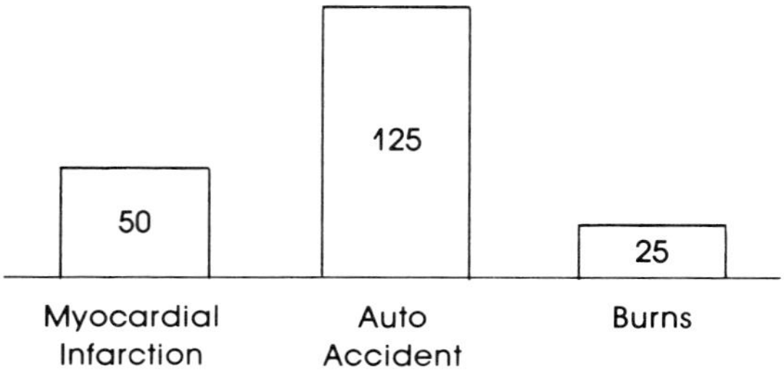

Figure 10–6. Bar graph. Number of patients admitted to an emergency room by diagnosis.

charts are often used to illustrate the breakdown of some quantity, like income, diagnosis, or age. When the percentages of various categories are converted to degrees of the circle, a pie chart clearly shows which slice indicates the largest category of the sample.

Bar Chart. A bar chart (shown in Figure 10–6) depicts frequencies for discontinuous categories, such as sex, occupation, or diagnosis. Bar charts can be presented either horizontally or vertically.

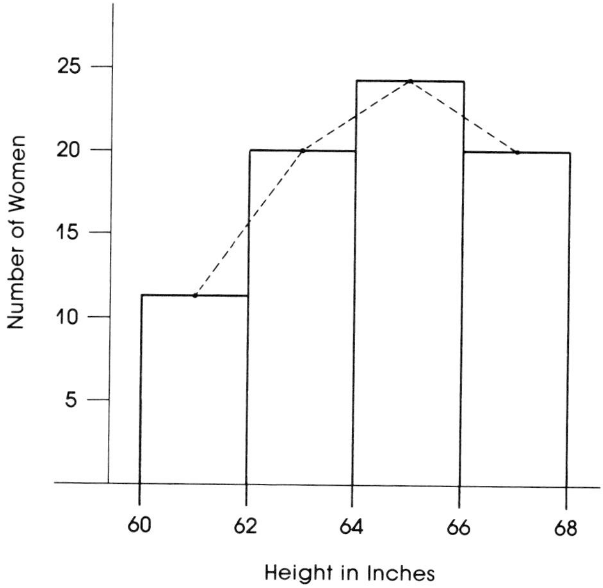

Figure 10–7. Histogram and frequency polygon used to depict a frequency distribution of height in a sample of women.

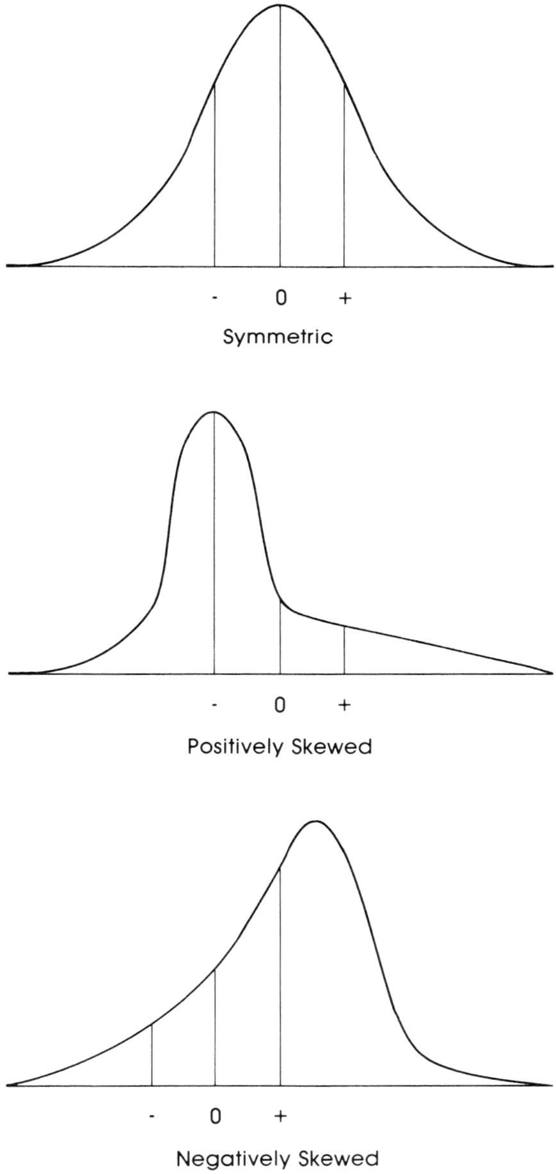

Figure 10–8. Examples of skewness.

Histogram. When a bar chart represents continuous data, the bars of data touch one another and the figure is called a histogram (shown in Figure 10–7).

Frequency Polygon. A frequency polygon, also illustrated in Figure 10–7, is constructed from a histogram by placing a dot in the center of the top of each bar and connecting these midpoints. A frequency polygon that has mirror-image shapes to the left and right of its middle is called *symmetrical*. However, when it is not a mirror image it is said to be *skewed* (shown in Figure 10–8). When the tail of the distribution is stretched out toward the high end of the scale it is *positively skewed*. The converse of a positively skewed frequency polygon is called *negatively skewed*.

ELEMENTS FOR CRITIQUE OF DATA ANALYSIS

- Are descriptive statistics used for all key variables?
- Is there evidence of non-normal distribution? That is, are standard deviations larger than the means?
- Are statistics appropriate to the level of measurement?
- Are statistical values reported?
- Are degrees of freedom reported?
- Are violations of underlying statistical assumptions addressed?
- Do the statistical procedures clarify, enhance, and address the research questions?
- Was the most effective statistic chosen?
- Was the level of significance reported?
- What consideration was given to Type I error?
- Was a bivariate procedure used when a multivariate procedure whould have been more appropriate?

Questions and Activities

1. *Describe the difference between a null hypothesis and a research hypothesis.*
2. *Compare parametric statistical assumptions with non-parametric assumptions.*
3. *Select a current issue of a nursing research journal. For each study reported, determine the statistical test(s) used.*
4. *For each of the above, determine how the statistical tests facilitated answering the research questions.*
5. *Why is it important to always report descriptive statistics?*
6. *Select a table from a current research study. Locate and identify its component parts.*

Bibliography

Cohen, I. B. (1984). Florence Nightingale. *Science, 250,* 128–137.

Greenwald, A. G. (1975). Consequences of prejudice against the null hypothesis. *Psychological Bulletin, 82,* 1–20.

Grier, B., and Grier, M. (1978). Contributions of the passionate statistician. *Research in Nursing and Health, 1,* 103–109.

Holm, K., and Christman, N. J. (1985). Post hoc tests following analysis of variance. *Research in Nursing and Health, 8,* 207–210.

Jalowiec, A., Murphy, S. P., and Powers, M. J. (1984). Psychometric assessment of the Jalowiec coping scale. *Nursing Research 33*(3), 157–161.

Krippendorff, K. (1980). *Content analysis: An introduction to its methodology.* Beverly Hills: Sage Publications.

Lamontagne, L. L. (1984). Children's locus of control beliefs as predictors of preoperative coping behavior. *Nursing Research, 33*(2), 76–79.

Leininger, M. (1984). Editorial. *Western Journal of Nursing Research, 6*(2), 151–152.

Powers, M. J., Murphy, S. P., and Wooldridge, P. J. (1983). Validation of two experimental nursing approaches using content analysis. *Research in Nursing and Health, 6,* 3–9.

Reid, B. J. (1983). Potential sources of type I error and possible solutions to avoid a "galloping" alpha rate. *Nursing Research, 32*(3), 190–191.

Siegel, S. (1956). *Nonparametric statistics for the behavioral sciences.* New York: McGraw-Hill.

Walker, H. M. (1940). Degrees of freedom. *Journal of Educational Psychology, 31,* 253–269.

Van Maanen, J. (1983). *Qualitative methodology.* Beverly Hills: Sage Publications.

11

Interpretation of Results

OBJECTIVES

After completing this chapter the reader will be able to:

1. Discuss factors involved in interpretation of results.
2. Address how findings should be integrated with previous work.
3. Discuss the relationship between research findings and conclusions.
4. Describe the significance of the power of a test.
5. Identify the role of recommendations for further research.

The introduction of a research report places the study problem within the context of current knowledge, while the interpretation of results identifies the extent to which contemporary knowledge has been expanded or extended by the research. Findings should be related to the work of others and should be explained in relation to purpose of the study.

CONSIDERATIONS IN THE INTERPRETATION OF RESULTS

Whether the results coincide with the purpose of the study is an important issue. Many times researchers get so involved in statistical tests, easily run by a computer, that they forget the original research questions. Such behavior leads to a discussion of results that is at best only somewhat related to the study's original intent.

The report and explanation of results of statistical tests must clearly relate to the research problem. Many times research reports appear with sophisticated statistical analyses that do not help to answer the research questions. Numbers can be easily entered into a computer program that produces a fancy output, but if the research question remains unanswered, such activity is without purpose.

Results are discussed in view of original expectations. If results coincide with expectations they are easier to explain, as the researcher has laid the groundwork in the introduction of the report. If results are in conflict with expectations, however, alternative explanations should be sought.

Other concerns are the methodological problems that may have influenced results. For example, if more than one person was involved in data collection, it is entirely possible that their approaches to data collection varied and that findings are consequently biased.

The subjects as well as the setting may also unduly influence findings. When, for example, subjects are aware that changes in policies or procedures are apt to be an outcome of a study, they may not respond to questions or interventions as they might have without the threat of change. Another consideration is whether the subjects were volunteers or were asked to participate following random selection. Random selection not only has implications for generalizability, that is, to what group or population of people can results be generalized, but decreases the probability of biased results due to sampling. Volunteers are self-selecting. They are people who are likely to enjoy participating in a study and may respond as they perceive a good subject should respond.

Another methodological issue likely to have an impact upon interpretation of results is the presence or absence of a control or comparison group. When statistically significant findings are interpreted without a comparison source, one is left to wonder, significant compared with whom or what? In addition, a small sample, missing data, or unequal group size can influence the outcomes of many statistical tests. So do extreme scores, sometimes referred to as outliers. A mean of 4.5 must be interpreted differently when it is the consequence of the addition of 6, 3, 4, and 5 as opposed to 14, 1, 2, and 1.

Interpreting data beyond what the numbers indicate is still another pitfall. Results must make logical sense. A good example of this is the researcher who interprets correlations in a cause-and-effect mode. For example, a finding that sub-zero temperatures are highly correlated with the incidence of heart attacks should not be interpreted as causal, specifically that an increase in heart attacks is directly caused by extreme cold. Another example occurs when an analysis of variance reveals significant differences but the researcher fails to use additional statistical tests (post hoc) to determine specifically where the significance lies.

INTEGRATION OF FINDINGS WITH PREVIOUS WORK

The findings of any study should not be interpreted in isolation. Findings must be integrated with previous research. In this section one expects to find how the present study supports or extends existing knowledge. There may also be findings that are in conflict with those previously documented. If contradictions do occur, there must be an attempt to explain or hypothesize the reason. In this situation the researcher may address the need for additional research based upon the fact that present findings depart substantially from existing knowledge. Before this is done, however, the researcher must demonstrate that attention was given to issues of internal validity such as controlling for the influences of history or maturation.

Table 11–1. TABLE SALT USE AND BLOOD PRESSURE

	Systolic	Diastolic
Low	123.9	76.9
Moderate	120.8	74.7
High	119.1	75.1

DRAWING CONCLUSIONS

Conclusions must be logical and appropriately fit the data from which they were drawn. Here again it is of essence that a researcher not go beyond the data. It may be easy to fall prey to such behavior when results are positive. A researcher excited about results may leap beyond what the data actually are indicating and draw inappropriate conclusions. It is true that many research journals prefer positive results, but editors and editorial boards are keenly aware of conclusions not supported by data.

Achieving statistical significance is not an end in itself. Investigators should also seek answers to questions of practical importance. Statistical significance suggests that results were probably real within the traditional 5 percent margin of error but indicates nothing about clinical significance. For example, a correlation of 0.17 significant at 0.01 due to a large sample size may be of little practical importance and be of little value in clinical practice.

This is particularly true when the size of the sample is large and even a small difference is statistically significant. Such was the case when Phillips and Holm (1985) classified 1078 people into three table salt use groups (low, moderate, high) and found that both systolic and diastolic pressures differed significantly among these groups. As shown in Table 11–1, the average pressures did not differ to any great extent and would not lead a clinician to radically alter a course of treatment. Yet for purposes of their study the differences suggested that table salt restriction may not be as important in the prevention of elevated blood pressures as national recommendations imply.

Non-significant results may lead to conclusions about the need to redesign a study because of methodological flaws such as confounding variables that may negate the impact of an experimental intervention. One may also conclude that negative or non-significant results offer an important contribution to clinical practice and are therefore of practical significance. In addition, lack of significant findings may be traced to the fact that concepts were not adequately measured or that a theoretical notion is incorrect. To reach such conclusions is in itself a contribution to science.

POWER OF A TEST

Even the most perfectly designed studies employing statistics correctly may fail at detecting significant or even clinically important differences simply because sample sizes are too small to give the statistic enough power to detect a difference. Statistical power is the ability of a statistical test to detect statistically significant differences when differences are present. The power of a statistical test is computed before the data are actually analyzed. The researcher specifies ahead of time (a priori) how small a change is worth detecting. Because this judgment is difficult to make, most investigators avoid power calculations. Yet such calculations can be very important, particularly in interpreting non-significant results. If one knows the power of a test to detect a significant difference is small, non-significant results may mean something different from the same results obtained from a more powerful test. Related to the power of a test is alpha or the risk of a Type I error. The difference between a Type I and a Type II error is shown in Table 11–2. To avoid committing a Type II error, a researcher increases the risk of a Type I error. But avoiding a Type II error, that is, not rejecting a false null

Table 11–2. TYPE I AND TYPE II ERROR

Type I	Rejecting a null hypothesis of equality when the null hypothesis is true. The risk of Type I error is designated alpha or level of significance.
Type II	Not rejecting a null hypothesis when it is false. The risk of Type II error is designated beta. Note that 1 − beta gives the power of a test.

hypothesis, may be more important. This is particularly true in clinical research, where even the most subtle experimental treatment effects must be identified.

RECOMMENDATIONS

The final section of a research report addresses recommendations for future research. This is the section that other investigators, both novice and experienced, should look to for guidance in the design of subsequent studies.

Investigators often address methodological issues or issues related to clinical practice. A common recommendation is that the present study be replicated using a larger sample size. Other recommendations that frequently appear include using a control or comparison group, using more sensitive measuring instruments, and securing a patient sample with a similar or dissimilar disease condition.

ELEMENTS FOR CRITIQUE OF INTERPRETATION OF RESULTS

- Are results interpreted in light of the original study problem?
- Do results coincide with expectations?
- Are results linked to previous research?
- Are results grounded in data?
- Are both negative and positive findings reported?
- Are weaknesses in the data honestly addressed?
- Are generalizations appropriate?
- Is practical significance addressed?
- Are conclusions justified?
- Are limitations clearly spelled out?
- What recommendations are made for implementation and further study?

In summary, recommendations for future research serve as a guide for studies that will follow. This part of a research report is quite valuable, as it identifies the direction that future research should take.

Questions and Activities

1. *Describe how a study can achieve statistical significance without being clinically significant.*
2. *What do you think about the tendency of some journals to avoid publishing studies with non-significant results?*
3. *How does the lack of a control group influence the conclusions of a study?*
4. *What are the possible conclusions that an investigator might make if a study's findings are not consistent with previous work in the area?*
5. *How is the power of a test related to Type II error?*

Bibliography

Levine, E. (1959). Interpreting statistical data. *American Journal of Nursing, 59,* 230–233.

Phillips, K., and Holm, K. (1985). Contemporary table salt use. *American Journal of Public Health, 74*(4), 405–406.

Weiner, E. E., and Weiner, D. L. (1983). Understanding the use of basic statistics in nursing research. *American Journal of Nursing, 83,* 770–774.

White, C. M. (1981). Presentation and interpretation of findings. In Y.M. Williamson (editor). *Research methodology and its application to nursing.* New York: John Wiley and Sons, 269–288.

Wilhite, M. J., and Unsain, I. C. (1979). Editorial: Statistical reporting: How accurate? How appropriate? *Nursing Research, 28*(5), 27.

V

PRACTICAL REALITIES OF RESEARCH

While the preceding units have dealt with the details of the research process, this unit addresses more practical issues and constraints of clinical research. Because dissemination of research findings is an acknowledged area of concern within the profession, the first chapter in this unit emphasizes the variety of ways in which research findings may be communicated. The next chapter focuses on the need to translate the findings into clinical practice. Following this discussion is a chapter related to ethical issues involved in human experimentation. The rights of subjects are emphasized and guidelines for their protection delineated. This unit concludes with acknowledgment of the real-world problems confronting the clinical nurse researcher and offers suggestions for their resolution.

12

Communicating Research

OBJECTIVES

After completing this chapter the reader will be able to:

1. Describe the types of written research reports.
2. Enumerate the desirable qualities of written research reports.

3. Summarize the relevant information to be included in each section of the report.
4. Describe outlets for oral presentations of research.

IMPORTANCE OF COMMUNICATING RESEARCH FINDINGS

The final step in the research process is communication of the findings. One's professional responsibility is not complete until the project is disseminated to professional colleagues. This communication can be oral, through presentations at seminars, clinical conferences, colloquia, and professional association meetings, or it can be written, as in a thesis, dissertation, abstract, or journal article.

It is desirable that a researcher choose several of these outlets for the same study so that results become more widely disseminated. For example, one can present a study at a conference, have its abstract published in the conference proceedings, and then write a more detailed report for a journal article.

TYPES OF WRITTEN RESEARCH REPORTS

Theses and Dissertations

A thesis or dissertation is a report of research conducted by a student in an academic program as a part of a degree requirement. (Thesis is the term generally used in relation to a master's degree, though not all master's programs require a formal thesis, and the term dissertation is more often used to describe the research report done for a doctoral degree.) It is important to remember that theses and dissertations are dual-purposed. Not only do they serve to communicate the findings of a scientific investigation, but more importantly, they serve to document the rigor and scholarship of a student's academic work. Thus, these documents tend to be much lengthier and more detailed than journal articles, providing very complete descriptions of the methods and a substantial review of the literature to demonstrate comprehensive understanding of the topic area.

Abstracts

An abstract is a brief summary of a research study that capsulizes the major points of the research findings. Often readers will skim the abstract to determine its relevance and then decide whether or not to read the entire study. Thus, an abstract may be the only part of a paper that is actually read by many people. (Of course, an informed research consumer will never stop with reading only the abstract, since erroneous conclusions may be drawn without the full details.)

Abstracts are generally 200 to 600 words in length. If there is a choice in the length of the abstract, shorter is usually preferable to longer. Abstracts are becoming increasingly significant with the trend toward computerized databases.

Journal Publications

Although many research conferences publish the abstracts of papers presented in a volume of proceedings, these do not ordinarily receive wide distribution, so researchers should also attempt to communicate to the larger community of nurses by reporting their studies in journals.

An increasing number of nursing journals are devoted primarily to publication of research studies (Table 12–1). However, nurses should not be strictly limited by research journals; many specialty journals now regularly include research reports. It is also important for nurses to publish in journals of other disciplines and even in the lay press.

The style (and even the content) of an article will depend upon the journal for which it is targeted. Other researchers are more likely

Table 12–1. NURSING JOURNALS WITH A RESEARCH EMPHASIS

Advances in Nursing Science	Journal of Professional Nursing
Communicating Nursing Research	Nursing Research
Image	Research in Nursing and Health
International Journal of Nursing Studies	Scholarly Inquiry for Nursing Practice
Journal of Advanced Nursing	Western Journal of Nursing Research

to be interested in the theoretical basis of the study and in the rigor of the methods, whereas an audience of clinical practitioners will probably be more interested in the results and what they mean for clinical practice. Once a potential journal has been selected, the author should skim several issues to get a flavor of the style and target level of the publication. It is also important to write to the editor to request that journal's author guidelines. (These are also published at the beginning of some journals.)

In McCloskey and Swanson's (1982) review of 100 nursing journals, editors were posed an open-ended question concerning advice that they would like to give to potential authors. Most of the editors who responded commented on the importance of knowing the journal. They emphasized being familiar with the journal audience and the purpose of the journal as well as reading the journal's information for contributors.

Ethics and professional courtesy demand that you not submit the same article simultaneously to more than one journal, although you may correspond with more than one editor if you wish. An example of a query letter to an editor is provided in Appendix I.

DESIRABLE QUALITIES FOR WRITTEN REPORTS

No amount of pretty packaging can disguise a poorly conceived project, but it is likely that an excellent project could go unnoticed or underestimated because of a report that is poorly organized, is incomplete, has confusing tables and graphs, or is loaded with jargon. Therefore, one should take as much care writing the report of the project as was put into the implementation of the project itself, keeping the following criteria in mind.

Clarity. Reports of research should be clearly written such that there can be no misinterpretation or guessing as to what was done in the project. Requesting review of a draft by colleagues and local experts can help to assure that the report conveys the essence of the study in a clear and straightforward, readable manner.

Precision. The research report should convey precisely and exactly the methods and results of the study. Avoid "weasel words" such as "maybe" and "possibly."

Honesty. A written research report should be an honest reflection of what occurred within the scope of the project. Researchers should not attempt to conceal mistakes or unintended consequences. On the contrary, it may be just such serendipitous occurrences that could be of greatest help to other researhers exploring the same subject. It goes without saying that hypotheses should not be changed nor data altered to "look good." The nature of science is putting one's work up for critique.

Brevity. Most journals are limited in space, necessitating that articles be presented in a brief, but complete, manner. Lengthy explanations and embellishments should be saved for other types of writing; they serve no useful purpose in a research report.

Completeness. Since another researcher should be able to read your report and replicate it under very similar conditions, this mandates that reports be complete. Inclusion of all important and relevant details of the study is important, not only for replication of the study, but so that others may more accurately critique the project and its outcomes.

Objectivity. Scientific writing demands objectivity. Most journals recommend the use of first person, although there is a recent trend toward making research reports more personal. Also, avoid adjectives such as "very" and "really."

Writing Style. Research reports are written in an objective, scholarly style. Unfortunately, this style is not familiar or comfortable for many nurses. Research writing is not literary writing. It is reporting of facts. Therefore, allegory, alliteration, poetic expressions, cliches, and lengthy embellishments are not appropriate. However, since scholarly is not the same thing as stuffy, research writing does not need to be dull or lifeless. Ideas should be presented in an interesting and compelling manner that reflects the author's involvement with the project.

Most journals now have policies regarding the use of non-sexist language in their publications. Wherever possible, male and female references should be avoided. Rewording and paraphrasing can usually result in sentences that do not specifically refer to gender. The *Publication Manual of the American Psychological Association* provides a nice summary of examples of how to avoid sex references. Although seemingly awkward at first, once one develops the habit of "neutral" writing, it will come naturally and will improve the overall quality of work in addition to minimizing the risk of inadvertently offending some readers.

WRITING EACH SECTION

The basic content of any written research report, whether it be a journal article or a dissertation, is similar and generally follows the same order as the research process. The major differences among the various forms of written reports lie only in the amount of detail included in each. The following is a summary of the relevant information to be included in each section of a written research report.

Title

Though it is often the element of a study that is given the least thought and attention, the title is a key concern. Many beginning researchers do not realize how important a title can be . Since a title is a study's window to the world, it should be interesting (in order to get people's attention) and complete (in order to convey the important elements of a study).

A researcher must make certain that the title includes all of the important key words related to the study's topic area, since this will be the key to indexing a study. Consulting a nursing thesaurus, such as the one in the *International Nursing Index*, may be helpful in pinpointing commonly used phrases or words.

Avoid obvious or redundant phrases in the title, such as "An Investigation to Examine the Effects of . . ." or "A Study of . . . ."

Introduction

The introduction tells the reader what was done and why; in other words, what was the point of the study? This section typically includes the statement of the problem and purpose, hypotheses, conceptual and operational definitions, and limitations and delimitations. It should also include the variables under consideration. Sometimes, if appropriate, the author may want to explain briefly how she became interested in the project.

Literature Review

The overall purpose of the literature review is to demonstrate the continuity between previous and present work. It also provides a theoretical rationale for the study.

In most studies an exhaustive historical review of the literature is not necessary. (The exception is doctoral dissertations, where this is sometimes expected so that the student demonstrates his or her knowledge of the background of the problem.) In other circumstances, the researcher should assume that the reader has a familiarity with the field and does not need all of the background studies. Reference to review articles is often helpful to give a broad overview.

Studies included in the review should be those that are directly related to the specific question under investigation. For example, if one is studying structured preoperative teaching in the coronary artery bypass graft (CABG) patient, one would include a summary of work relating to structured teaching in general and studies of teaching with CABG patients and perhaps related patient groups, such as post–myocardial infarction patients. Studies of teaching and learning principles involved in unstructured teaching with unrelated patient populations would not be appropriate to include unless directly related to the problem or methods.

Methods

The methods section tells the reader the details of how the study was conducted. By reading the methods section, a reader should be able to learn how to replicate the study reasonably well. The methods section consists of the following subsections:

Overview. One or two comprehensive paragraphs should outline the overall approach to the conduct of the study. This gives the reader a "thumbnail sketch" of the project. Sometimes this section includes a diagram of the research design, especially if it is experimental or quasi-experimental.

Setting. The setting is described so that the reader can judge whether or not the study was conducted in a place that allowed for sufficient control of the variables. It also includes any environmental conditions that may have influenced the study's results.

Subjects. This section, also sometimes called "sample," answers the questions: Who participated in the study? How many participants were there? How were they selected? The writer should make clear the population to whom the results might be generalized and how the sample from that population was drawn. It is also expected that you mention subjects who did not participate in the study and whether they differed in any characteristic ways from those who did. This section sometimes includes the method for ensuring subjects' rights, such as privacy and consent, although some reports will include this as a separate section.

Instruments. This section describes any tools or instruments that were used in data collection. If they are original, it describes how they were developed and pre-tested. It also includes information about the validity and reliability of the instruments. Either sample questions are provided or sometimes the entire instrument may be reproduced in a table or in an appendix. When bioinstrumentation is used, the specifications should be included.

Data Collection. Also sometimes called "procedure," this section details the steps followed in the execution of the research. This section tells what you did and *how* you did it. If there were any problems in following the originally planned methods, they should be discussed briefly here. No study is perfect, and investigators should be open and honest about any modifications that may have been necessary in the course of the project.

Findings

The findings or "results" section gives a summary of the data and the statistical treatment and results. There are several ways of organizing this section. Many researchers begin with descriptive findings regarding the sample and its equivalence on key variables. A logical way of organizing the remainder of this section is by hypotheses, explaining the first hypothesis, the test of it, and the results of the test, then the second, and so on. Usually the results section is merely an objective reporting of what was found without judgment or interpretation; the discussion and elaboration of the findings is usually saved for a following section.

Clarification of the results is enhanced by the inclusion of summary statistics, either in the body of the paper or within tables, figures, and graphs. The writer needs to be careful, however, not to needlessly duplicate information in text and tables. Tables should enhance understanding of the findings rather than merely repeat them. Be aware, however, that tables and graphs are expensive to reproduce, and therefore many publishers advise authors to limit their use.

The researcher does not necessarily report all of the analyses that were performed. If they are tangential and do not bear relation to the problem under study, they should not be mentioned, just as the review of literature does not include every single article read by the author.

Be careful when reporting statistical findings to use words with precise statistical meaning only as they are exactly intended. A common mistake is to speak of a relation or correlation in "generic" terms when no actual correlational statistics were used, or to talk of "significance" when the intent is "importance."

Discussion, Conclusions, and Recommendations

The results section tells what happened, but the discussion attempts to shed light on why it happened. This section is the researcher's opportunity to pull the study together, showing connections and relationships.

Answer the following questions: Did I answer the research question, and how was it answered? What have I contributed? How has my study helped to resolve the original problem? What conclusions and theoretical implications can I draw from my study? What recommendations can I make to others regarding this problem? Comparison and contrast with previous work should be evident. Acknowledge flaws and limitations in the study but do not dwell on them. Cautious speculation is allowed, but one should be careful not to generalize beyond the scope of the study.

References

People often misunderstand the difference between references and a bibliography. References are those materials intended to give credence to the subject under study. They are actually cited in the report. On the other hand, a bibliography contains materials used only to give a background preparation needed for the study.

References have been likened to vitamin consumption; if one is good, multiplying the dose is not necessarily better (Downs, 1980). References should be kept to a minimum, particularly in journal articles. The writer should retain only enough so that an educated reader would be able to understand the importance of the investigation and how it relates to other work, and to explicate the theoretical rationale.

It is best to use the strongest and most recent references. Avoid unpublished works when possible; they are rarely pivotal works. Older but seminal work is not considered dated and should be included. It is permissible to refer to review articles to document the state of the art, but one should return to the original source for any actual data that are to be used.

COLLOQUIUM AND SYMPOSIUM PRESENTATIONS

Local, regional, and national meetings are also good outlets for the communication of nursing research. Oral presentation of a study has two clear advantages over the written report. First, oral presentations can almost always be accomplished sooner than publication in a journal. Thus, findings are disseminated more rapidly. Secondly, because the presentation is face-to-face with others, there is opportunity for exchange of ideas. The audience can request clarification and expansion of points, and the researcher has the advantage of being able to get feedback from other practitioners and researchers.

Calls for papers for conferences and symposia can be found in many nursing journals. If your research is related to a specific clinical specialty, you might want to look in that specialty's journals for upcoming meetings that might be appropriate for the presentation of your work.

The format for a paper presented at a conference is similar to that of a written report and generally follows the same order. However, since most conferences allow only 20 to 30 minutes for presentation, the content of the report must be considerably reduced, highlighting only the major points of the study. Since only the most important aspects can be highlighted, it is helpful to use slides to enhance the audience's understanding of the details of the study. A listener cannot follow the same level of detail as a reader.

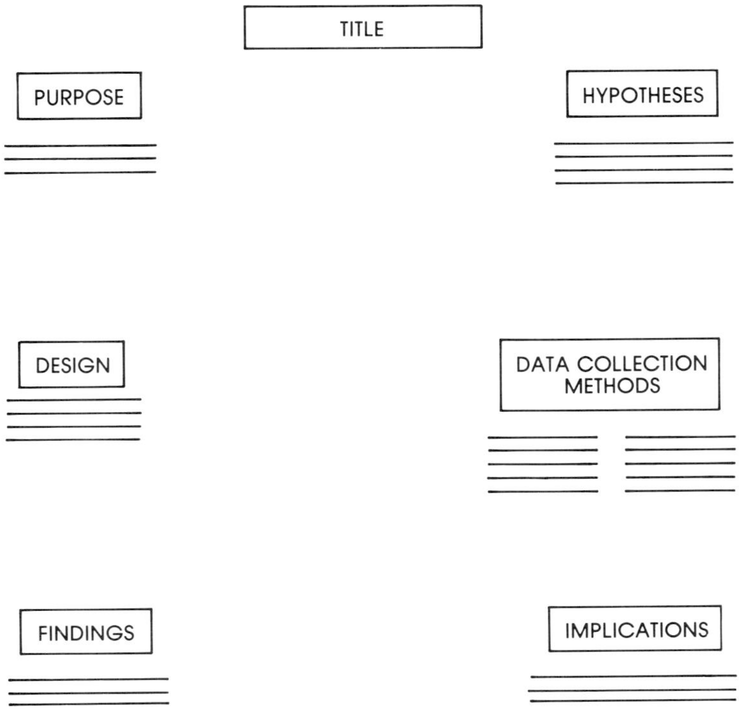

Figure 12–1. Suggested layout for a typical research poster.

POSTER SESSIONS

At a poster session, a researcher is given an area (often 4 feet by 6 feet) and a table upon which to display her research visually. The poster may be accompanied by supplemental materials, such as samples of instruments or even audiovisual aids. The popularity of poster sessions is increasing, probably owing to their informal atmosphere and the opportunity that is afforded for discussion and feedback from colleagues.

It is sometimes helpful to use graph paper in making a scale model of your exhibit. By so doing, you can make certain your charts and photographs will fit into the space allotted. It will also help you to better organize the overall presentation as you arrange and rearrange the components. Figure 12–1 illustrates one suggested arrangement for a typical poster.

Keep the amount of information presented to a minimum. Excessive information will not impress viewers to the point where they will say "It looks like you've been working hard," as much as they will tend to say "What a mess!" In order to communicate more

ELEMENTS FOR CRITIQUE OF REPORT OF RESULTS

- Does the title of the study reflect key variables?
- Is there a clearly stated, brief abstract?
- Is the report logically organized?
- Is the bibliography related to the central theme?
- Is there clear documentation of others' work?
- Is the format consistent throughout?
- Has the investigator been honest in reporting results?
- Is the study reported in sufficient detail to allow replication?
- Is the report written in a professional style?
- Is non-sexist language used?
- Are tables, graphs, and charts used to enhance text?
- Is the report written in an interesting manner?

detailed information about a project, many poster presenters also have copies of their abstracts available for distribution to participants.

Questions and Activities

1. *Examine a current issue of a clinical nursing journal. Determine which articles seem to be based on research findings.*
2. *Using current professional journals, identify meetings and conferences where nursing research might be presented.*
3. *How might a thesis or dissertation differ from a journal article?*
4. *What are the advantages of poster sessions?*
5. *Why is it important for nurse researchers to publish in the lay press in addition to publishing in the professional literature?*

Bibliography

Binger, J. L. (1979). Writing for publication: A survey of nursing journal editors. *Journal of Nursing Administration*, 9, 50–52.

Day, R. A. (1979). *How to write and publish a scientific paper*. Philadelphia: ISI Press.

Downs, F. S. (1980). Wielding Occam's razor. *Nursing Research*, *29*(5), 269.

Fawcett, J. (1984). Communicating research findings: Oral presentations. *Reflections*, *10*, 2.

Kolin, P. C., and Kolin, J. L. (1980). *Professional writing for nurses in education, practice, and research*. St. Louis: C.V. Mosby.

Maxwell, M. (1980). The agony and the ecstasy: How to successfully write and publish your paper. *Oncology Nursing Forum*, *7*(3), 41–47.

McCloskey, J. C., and Swanson, E. (1982). Publishing opportunities for nurses: A comparison of 100 journals. *Image*, *14*(2), 50–56.

Mirin, S. K. (1981). *The nurses's guide to writing for publication*. Wakefield, MA: Nursing Resources.

Morra, M. (1984). How to plan and carry out your poster session. *Oncology Nursing Forum*, *11*, 52–57.

Robinson, A., and Notter, L. (1982). *Clinical writing*. Bowie, MD: Robert Brady Co.

Sexton, D. L. (1984). Presentation of research findings: The poster session. *Nursing Research*, *33*(6), 374–375.

Strunk, W., and White, E. B. (1979). *The elements of style*. 3rd edition. New York: Macmillan.

Styles, M. M. (1978). Why publish? *Image*, *10*(2), 28–32.

Swanson, E., and McCloskey, J. C. (1982). The manuscript review process of nursing journals. *Image, 14*(3), 72–76.

Tornquist, E. M. (1983). Strategies for publishing research. *Nursing Outlook, 31*(3), 180–183.

Werley, H. H., Murphy, P. A., Gosch, S. M., Gottesmann, H., and Newcomb, B. J. (1981). Research publication credit assignment: Nurses' views. *Research in nursing and health, 4*, 261–279.

13

Research Utilization

OBJECTIVES

After completing this chapter the reader will be able to:

1. Describe barriers to the implementation of nursing research findings.
2. Describe the role of the administrator, researcher, and clinician in fostering a research climate.

The field of nursing research reads like familiar "good news/bad news" stories. The good news is that nursing research is flourishing. Signs of life on several fronts are promising: research courses in curricula of colleges of nursing are standard; the volume of nursing research increases each year; conferences and symposia for the purposes of communicating research are commonplace; centers and departments of nursing research are being established not only at the major universities, but in smaller programs and in clinical facilities as well; several scholarly research-based nursing journals enjoy success; increased numbers of nurses hold graduate degrees; increased numbers of nurses have earned doctorates; and nurses compete successfully with other scientists for research dollars.

The bad news is that the fruits of nursing research are agonizingly slow in becoming incorporated into everyday clinical practice. The dissemination of findings lags far behind the completion of studies. In a recent survey (Stokes, 1981) it was determined that research findings had little effect on current nursing practice by nurses in that sample. Further, validation of research findings through replication of studies is uncommon.

This problem tends to compound itself in a circular, self-defeating manner. If relevant research is not generated and used by practitioners, further research is discouraged. If results are not implemented, they cannot be evaluated. Researchers do not receive feedback and remain ignorant of the utility of their work, and practitioners remain skeptical. The cycle feeds on itself and perpetuates a non-productive situation.

In this chapter, the dilemma of research utilization will be explored. Barriers to the implementation of research findings into clinical practice will be discussed, and suggestions for fostering a climate for research utilization will be proposed.

BARRIERS TO THE IMPLEMENTATION OF NURSING RESEARCH FINDINGS

Failure of Researchers to Communicate Their Findings to Practitioners. Much of the research conducted by nurses goes unpublished. How many master's theses and doctoral dissertations remain sitting on the shelf, known only to the student and a small faculty committee?

How many small clinical studies remain confined to a single institution's use? A beginning step in research utilization is to assure that studies are shared with nursing colleagues. Any study worth doing is worth doing well, and any study worth doing well is worth reporting.

Regarding research that is reported, the unfortunate fact is that most research is reported by nurse researchers to other nurse researchers. Researchers communicate with each other, not with clinicians. Most staff nurses do not subscribe to research journals, nor do they usually attend research conferences. Conversely, researchers do not ordinarily take their studies into the clinical practice arena.

When researchers and practitioners do get together, a further problem is that they do not speak the same language. Communication between the two is blocked because of the excessive use of jargon and technical terminology.

Chasm Between Education, Research, and Practice. Most nursing research is done in institutions of higher education, yet most practitioners are in service settings. Their paths seldom cross, and thus there have evolved two subcultures, as Ketefian (1975) has suggested. Furthermore, nursing faculty, unlike their counterparts in most other professional disciplines, are not generally engaged in their own practice and research, so students are not exposed to credible behavioral models and thus do not develop strong research values. A related problem is that when researchers are so far removed from clinical practice, they are less likely to pose the important clinical questions. Research in such an environment lacks the depth and richness that is possible when research, practice, and education are wedded.

Lack of Theoretical Cohesiveness of Nursing Research. Although an increasing volume of research is being conducted, much of it remains as isolated bits without a strong bond to a central area of investigation. There is a lack of conceptually related research upon which to confidently base clinical interventions. Similarly, there is minimal replication of studies to confirm or validate the research being produced, or to validate and expand the findings of the many small pilot studies conducted.

Confusion Among Practitioners Regarding the Differences Between the Conduct of Research and the Utilization of Research. Horsley and Crane (1983), in their experience in the project titled Conduct and Utilization of Research in Nursing (CURN), have observed through experience on the project that nurses often confuse the conduct of research with the utilization of research findings. They cite as an example the fact that when asked to describe how they might use research in their practice, nurses often described a process of replication. Horsley and Crane further delineated the differences in the goals of each: *research conduct* is directed toward the production of knowledge that is generalizable beyond the population directly studied, whereas *research utilization* is directed toward transferring specific research-based knowledge into actual practice.

Differences in Methodology Between Research and Practice. Although the scientific method and nursing process share many similarities and one has grown out of the other, basic differences in the tenets of the scientific method are in sharp contrast to the methodologies commonly used in clinical practice. The methods of research are systematic, controlled, and generally inflexible. Research is rigorous and there are attempts to minimize personal bias. On the other hand, clinical methods rely heavily on skill and are individualized. They are relatively flexible, may rely on precedent, and draw upon clinical judgment. The nurse in clinical practice tends to take an intuitive approach and regards each case as unique.

Haller, Reynolds, and Horsley (1979) view these differences as important because they affect the interactions that occur between nurses in the research and practice settings. They propose that both groups need to begin to learn each other's approaches in order to close the gap between research methods and practice methods.

Studies' Lack of Relevance to Practice. If nursing studies do not address a nursing problem in a clinical setting, they will likely not be of interest to practitioners. Unfortunately, many nursing studies either are not relevant or are one or more steps removed from being directly applicable to clinical practice.

The CURN project suggested that a study's degree of relevance to clinical practice may be judged by four criteria: (1) degree of clinical merit, (2) extent of clinical control over the variables, (3) feasibility, and (4) cost.

Disparity in Level of Educational Preparation of Nurses. While all nurses have a mandate to increase and utilize the scientific base for clinical practice, the reality within the profession is that most nurses in clinical practice do not possess the educational preparation necessary to perform or evaluate formal investigative activities. Many nursing education programs below the baccalaureate level include no research preparation at all. It is not surprising that many nurses lack basic research knowledge and do not understand the language of research.

Nonetheless, nurses prepared at any educational level have a role to play in developing scientific knowledge and incorporating that knowledge into practice. No single group of nurses should be expected to shoulder the responsibility of building a scientific base for professional practice. The Commission on Nursing Research of the American Nurses' Association has recommended investigative functions for nurses consistent with educational preparation. They are listed in Table 13–1.

Institutional Barriers to Change. Even when practitioners have the knowledge and motivation to conduct, implement, and utilize research, often institutional and administrative barriers prohibit research utilization. Nurses may find the bureaucratic structure too overwhelmingly cumbersome to attempt to institute changes in practice based upon investigative findings. The institution may not value research at all and may discourage research by not providing time for it, by not rewarding it, and by holding rigidly to policy and procedure, rather than by being open to data-based evolving clinical practices. Another organizational factor that inhibits research utilization is evident when practitioners are allowed minimal decision-making authority regarding their practice. Thus, even if a clinician does discover a data-based solution to a problem, if she is not allowed the autonomy to implement it, then it will not likely be reflected in practice.

FOSTERING A CLIMATE FOR RESEARCH UTILIZATION

Mauksch (1973) suggests that we need to develop a research climate:

> that means a work climate which is not exclusive, but inclusive; one which is not restrictive, but is open. That means the provision of a great variety of positive supportive behaviors on the part of us all. Regardless of whether we are researchers, practitioners, teachers, or administrators, if we function

Table 13–1. GUIDELINES FOR THE INVESTIGATIVE FUNCTION OF NURSES*

Associate Degree in Nursing

1. Demonstrates awareness of the value or relevance of research in nursing.
2. Assists in identifying problem areas in nursing practice.
3. Assists in collection of data within an established structured format.

Baccalaureate in Nursing

1. Reads, interprets, and evaluates research for applicability to nursing practice.
2. Identifies nursing problems that need to be investigated and participates in the implementation of scientific studies.
3. Uses nursing practice as a means of gathering data for refining and extending practice.
4. Applies established findings of nursing and other health-related research to nursing practice.
5. Shares research findings with colleagues.

Master's Degree in Nursing

1. Analyzes and reformulates nursing practice problems so that scientific knowledge and scientific methods can be used to find solutions.
2. Enhances the quality and clinical relevance of nursing research by providing expertise in clinical problems and by providing knowledge about the way in which these clinical services are delivered.
3. Facilitates investigations of problems in clinical settings through such activities as contributing to a climate supportive of investigative activities, collaborating with others in investigations and enhancing nursing's access to clients and data.
4. Conducts investigations for the purpose of monitoring the quality of the practice of nursing in a clinical setting.
5. Assist others to apply scientific knowledge in nursing practice.

Doctoral Degree in Nursing or a Related Discipline

A. Graduate of a practice-oriented doctoral program
   1. Provides leadership for the integration of scientific knowledge with other sources of knowledge for the advancement of practice.
   2. Conducts investigations to evaluate the contribution of nursing activities to the well-being of clients.
   3. Develops methods to monitor the quality of the practice of nursing in a clinical setting and to evaluate contributions of nursing activities to the well-being of clients.

B. Graduate of a research-oriented doctoral program
   1. Develops theoretical explanations of phenomena relevant to nursing by empirical research and analytical processes.
   2. Uses analytical and empirical methods to discover ways to modify or extend existing scientific knowledge so that it is relevant to nursing.
   3. Develops methods for scientific inquiry of phenomena relevant to nursing

*This language was developed as part of the work of the ANA Commission on Nursing Education and was included in the report of that commission to the 1980 ANA House of Delegates.

From Commission on Nursing Research (1981). *Guidelines for the investigative function of nurses.* Kansas City, MO: Amertican Nurses' Association.

in a setting where nursing practice occurs, we must learn to impart to those around us our enthusiasm and our commitment to the research process.

Though development of a favorable research climate is a difficult task, when individual practitioners, administrators, and researchers undertake a concerted effort, their results can be fruitful. Specific ways each level can contribute to creating such a favorable climate will be described in the following sections.

CLINICIAN-LEVEL INDIVIDUAL ACCOUNTABILITY

The mystique surrounding the word "research" must be removed before research will be successfully incorporated into the everyday realm of clinical nursing practice. Individual practitioners must come to realize that research does not need to be a highly formalized and formidable undertaking; in reality, the management of each patient involves investigative activity.

In fact, most nurses possess many of the skills needed to critique and use research; being an intelligent consumer of research is not unlike being an intelligent consumer of goods and services (Mayo and LaFrance, 1977). A good consumer knows the necessity of reading labels and packages carefully; similarly, a conscientious consumer of research knows to evaluate a study on the basis of the "fine print" of the methodology, realizing that results are only as good as the methods used to obtain them. Other consumer skills that are equally applicable to the consumption of research include: checking guarantees (seeing that the conclusions are not generalized beyond the actual results); looking beyond flashy merchandizing (making sure the outcome matches the research question); and assessing durability (determining generalizability). When nurses realize that research is not something to be feared but something to be utilized in improving their own practice, then the mystique of research will dwindle and research utilization will increase.

Research utilization is a professional responsibility at any level of clinical practice. In outlining investigative functions of nurses, the Commission on Nursing Research of the American Nurses' Association has stated:

To maximize the benefits of developing a scientific base for use in practice, mechanisms are required that ensure that scientific knowledge contributes to practice and in turn that the problems encountered in practice have an impact on the focus of the knowledge generated. Nurses performing different roles in nursing contribute to the interplay between practice and research that builds the scientific base for practice. Identification of types of involvement expected from nurses performing the various roles is essential to building a scientific base for nursing practice.

Not every nurse needs to be a full-fledged investigator, but until all nurses value scientific inquiry as a means to solve patient management problems, research utilization in the clinical arena will continue to flounder. It is clear that nurses will be unable to support research utilization if the behaviors expected of them are not clearly outlined and communicated. In addition, these behaviors must be realistically within their potential to fulfill, should be tangibly rewarded, and should be administratively supported. A clinical ladder or a levels of practice system that includes research activities is a helpful mechanism whereby this can occur. Table 13–2 demonstrates one such approach.

Through mechanisms such as these, it may be possible that research will become an internalized part of the full professional role for nurses as it has become in other more fully developed professions. When the average practicing nurse assumes that research is an integral part of practice, then the value of research will have been integrated and incorporated into professional thinking and research utilization will be the standard in nursing.

ADMINISTRATOR-LEVEL ORGANIZATIONAL ACCOUNTABILITY

Administrative support for research utilization involves creating a climate whereby communication of research information is facilitated and implementation of findings is possible. If the organization can also provide supports for the actual conduct of research, then that is all the better. Table 13–3 summarizes one approach to delineating research activities at various administrative levels.

Table 13–2. RESEARCH EXPECTATIONS OF STAFF NURSES ACCORDING TO LEVELS

Level A (Beginning Practitioner)	Level B (Experienced Clinical Nurse)	Level C (Expert Clinical Nurse)
Cooperates in applying research findings to patient care.	Applies concepts from current health reports to patient care.	Introduces concepts from health care research for application in the clinical setting.
Assists with identifying patient care problems for investigation.	Identifies problems in the clinical practice of nursing which are suitable for investigation.	Assists with staff development and implementation of nursing and health-related studies.
Cooperates in collecting data for research projects.	Participates in critically evaluating existing nursing practice.	Serves as a resource for interdisciplinary research.
	Evaluates the effectiveness of new methods and communicates outcome.	

Adapted from Rush–Presbyterian–St. Luke's Medical Center, Chicago, IL, Levels of Nursing Practice system.

An organizational structure that has the strongest likelihood of fostering research implementation is one in which research, education, and clinical practice are all within one management structure. When these aspects are wedded, many of the barriers to research utilization—such as access to ideas, communication of a value system, delineation of relevant questions, and research resources—are much easier to overcome.

In more traditional administrative structures, there is still much that can be done from a management level to promote research utilization. Practitioners cannot use knowledge they don't have, so efforts to promote the communication of research are essential. This can be done through such mechanisms as journal clubs, grand rounds, research bulletins, and other similar means. When access is not available within the organization, then support for sending practitioners to outside conferences and a mechanism for them to report back to their colleagues should be facilitated.

A system of clinical advancement (levels of practice) in which practitioners are rewarded for research utilization activities should

Table 13–3. RESEARCH EXPECTATIONS OF ADMINISTRATIVE STAFF

Head Nurse	Clinical Faculty	Quality Assurance
Assists with planning, implementing, or evaluating studies, projects, or research activities.	Plans and implements studies and projects.	Collects data for the monitoring of the quality of nursing care.
Encourages and interprets solutions to problems through research methods	Encourages nursing staff to seek solutions to problems through research.	Participates in the design and implementation of special studies regarding the quality of care.
Clinical Chair/Chief/Director		
Participates in implementation of studies and projects.		
Promotes departmental research.		
Interprets research projects and/or findings to nursing staff.		
Collaborates with members of related disciplines in research activities.		
Prepares grant proposals; seeks funding.		
Reviews outside requests for research approval.		

Adapted from Rush–Presbyterian–St. Lukes's Medical Center, Chicago, IL, Levels of Nursing Practice system.

be encouraged. Managers should also look for other less formal ways by which research utilization can be recognized, rewarded, and thereby valued in the organization.

Another crucial factor for a favorable research environment is supporting the value of seeking answers to clinical dilemmas through formal investigation. This attitude can be communicated through mechanisms such as the policy and procedure committee by helping members to assure that all policies and procedures are data-based. When clinical questions arise, managers can encourage nurses to investigate research solutions and make resources available for research. In addition, educational departments can address current research findings in their continuing education programs.

All of these efforts toward research utilization will be futile, however, if nurses do not have autonomy and control over their own practice. If their nursing actions are governed by the wishes of others, then it will be inevitable that their attempts to change practice will be thwarted. A structure in which primary nursing is the mode of care delivery enhances individual practitioners' autonomy, and a self-governance structure for the nursing staff further ensures control over issues of nursing practice.

Nurse managers can also create learning experiences whereby potential researchers can work with more experienced investigators to develop the needed skills. Nurses come from a tradition of apprenticeship, so this can be a natural way for novices to gain experience.

RESEARCHER-LEVEL PROFESSIONAL ACCOUNTABILITY

One of the first steps in improving research utilization must be the clear communication of research findings to clinical practitioners. Researchers must share the responsibility for reporting, both verbally and through the professional literature, the findings of their investigations. These reports must be presented in clear, understandable language, free from excessive jargon and technical terminology. Furthermore, until the average nurse becomes proficient in critiquing and interpreting research findings, researchers will also need to be interpreters, extrapolating the important clinical implications and pointing them out to practitioners.

This communication ought also to extend beyond the professional bounds of the discipline of nursing. Knowledge gained through nursing research should be shared widely with other disciplines and with the lay population, since it is not only nurses who will utilize nursing knowledge.

Another responsibility of the clinical researcher is to be involved with clinical practice. If an investigator intends to do clinical research, there is an attendant obligation to be sufficiently cognizant of the practice arena to be able to ask cogent questions. One method to ensure that researchers consider specific practice application of studies is to require that a plan for utilization be a central part of the proposal stage. Unless concepts are empirically referenced in practice, clinical research will continue to be one or more steps beyond what is needed in the real world of patients.

Questions and Activities

1. *List the barriers to the implementation of nursing research findings and suggest strategies to overcome them.*
2. *How can a clinical ladder facilitate research utilization?*
3. *As a clinician, what steps do you plan to take to utilize nursing research findings in your area of interest?*
4. *Refer to the "Guidelines for the Investigative Function of Nurses" published by the American Nurses' Association. Do you agree or disagree?*
5. *Review a current issue of a research journal. Suggest ways in which the reported findings might be used in clinical practice.*

Bibliography

Butts, P. A. (1982). Dissemination of nursing research findings. *Image, 14*(2), 62–64.

Castles, M. B. (1975). A practitioner's guide to utilization of research findings. *Journal of Obstetric and Gynecologic Nursing, 4*(1), 50–53.

Commission on Nursing Research (1981). *Guidelines for the investigative function of nurses.* Kansas City, MO: American Nurses' Association.

Crane, J. (1980). Factors influencing research utilization in nursing practice. *Communicating Nursing Research, 13,* 36–37.

Crane, J. (1985). Research utilization: Theoretical perspectives. *Western Journal of Nursing Research, 7*(2), 261–268.

Engstrom, J. L. (1984). University, agency, and collaborative models for nursing research: An overview. *Image, 16*(3), 76–80.

Fawcett, J. (1982). Utilization of nursing research findings. *Image, 14*(2), 57–59.

Fawcett, J. (1984). Another look at utilization of nursing research. *Image, 16*(2), 59–62.

Feldman, H. R. (1980). Nursing research in the 1980s: Issues and implications. *Advances in Nursing Sciences, 3*(1), 85–92.

Haller, K. B., Reynolds, M. A., and Horsley, J. A. (1979). Developing research-based innovation protocols: Process, criteria, and issues. *Research in Nursing and Health, 2,* 45–51.

Hefferin, E. A., Horsley, J. A., and Ventura, M. R. (1982). Promoting research-based nursing: The nurse administrator's role. *Journal of Nursing Administration, 12,* 34–41.

Horsley, J., and Crane, J. (1983). *Using research to improve nursing practice: A guide.* New York: Grune and Stratton.

Horsley, J. A. (1985). Using research in practice: The current context. *Western Journal of Nursing Research, 7*(1), 135–139.

Jacobs, M. K.,and Huether, S. E. (1978). Nursing science: The theory-practice linkage. *Advances in Nursing Science, 1*(1), 63–73.

Jacox, A. (1980), Strategies to promote nursing research. *Nursing Research, 29*(4), 213–217.

Ketefian, S. (1975). Application of selected nursing research findings into nursing practice: A pilot study. *Nursing Research, 24*(2), 89–92.

Kirchhoff, K. T. (1983). Using research in practice: Should staff nurses be expected to use research? *Western Journal of Nursing Research, 5*, 245–247.

Krone, K. P., and Loomis, M. E. (1982). Developing practice-relevant research: A model that worked. *Journal of Nursing Administration, 12*, 38–41.

Krueger, J. (1977). Utilizing clinical nursing research findings in practice: A structured approach. *Communicating Nursing Research, 9*, 381–394.

Lindeman, C. A. (1984). Dissemination of nursing research. *Image, 16*(2), 57–58.

Loomis, M. E. (1985). Knowledge utilization and research utilization in nursing. *Image, 17*(2), 35–39.

Mauksch, I. G. (1973). Social responsibilities of the nurse scientist. In *Issues in research: Social, professional, and methodological*. Selected papers from the ANA Council of Nurse Researchers program meeting, Kansas City, MO, 2–8.

Mayo, C., and LaFrance, M. (1977). *Evaluation research in social psychology: A guide for the consumer*. Monterey, CA: Brooks/Cole.

Mercer, R. T. (1984). Nursing research: The bridge to excellence in practice. *Image, 16*(2), 47–51.

Miller, J. R., and Messenger, S. R. (1978). Obstacles to applying nursing research findings. *American Journal of Nursing, 78*(4), 632–634.

Paletta, J. L. (1980), Nursing research: An integral part of professional nursing. *Image, 12*, 3–6.

Stetler, C. B., and Marram, G. (1976). Evaluating research findings for applicability in practice. *Nursing Outlook, 24*, 559–563.

Stevenson, J. S. (1978). Developing staff research potential: Part one. *Journal of Nursing Administration, 8*(5), 44–46.

Stevenson, J. S. (1978). Developing staff research potential: Part two: Planning and implementation of studies. *Journal of Nursing Administration, 8*(6), 8–12.

Stokes, J. E. (1981). Utilization of research findings by staff nurses. In S. D. Krampitz and N. Pavlovich (editors). *Readings for nursing research* (pp. 227–234). St. Louis: C. V. Mosby.

14

Practical Considerations in the Ethics of Human Investigations

OBJECTIVES

After completing this chapter the reader will be able to:

1. Describe historical events that led to the concern for research ethics.
2. List the basic principles included in the major ethical codes.
3. Describe the elements of informed consent.
4. Describe assessment of risk-benefit ratio.

5. Anticipate concerns when research is conducted within the context of the helping relationship.
6. Differentiate between the types of research review.
7. Describe ethical concerns when investigating populations at risk.

ETHICS IN RESEARCH—AN OVERVIEW

Research with human beings is essential from a utilitarian standpoint since some research questions are answerable only when studied in human subjects. However, owing to the astonishing abuse of subjects in research within our lifetimes, questions are raised about the immediate and long-term consequences upon human lives. Are short-term risks to individuals justified by the potential for positive consequences for the greater number of people? Do the ends justify the means? Such questions are at the heart of discussions of research ethics.

Before World War II, the ethics of research and experimentation with humans was unregulated and went largely undiscussed. However, during the Nuremberg trials of World War II Nazi war criminals, many atrocities committed in the name of research were exposed. The world was horrified to hear of sterilizations, dissections of the brain and heart of living people, lethal injections of typhus, and freezing experiments, to name a few. These testimonies led to a large-scale raising of the world consciousness regarding the potential dangers of human experimentation.

Within the United States prior to 1962, the medical research community exercised individual personal and professional judgment as to the ethical conduct of research. However, two landmark events marked the beginning of federal regulation of research.

Both of these occurrences involved research in the area of pharmaceuticals. First were the tragedies resulting from the testing of thalidomide, in which large numbers of infants were born with severe birth defects as a result of inadequate testing of a drug. The second significant event to influence federal regulation was the Kefauver congressional investigation of the drug industry. For more than two years, Senator Estes Kefauver conducted hearings concerning the testing and marketing of drugs during which flagrant ethical violations were exposed.

As a result of these and other factors, laws were passed in 1962 that subjected any drug studies to regulations administered by the Food and Drug Administration. A few years later, in 1966, it became a requirement that all Public Health Service grants be reviewed by a committee at the sponsoring institution.

However, the most broad-reaching legislation was passed in 1974 with the enactment of Public Law 93–348, the National Research Act. This act established the National Commission for the Protection of Human Subjects of Biomedical and Behavioral Research. This commission was mandated to "identify the basic ethical principles which should underlie the conduct of biomedical and behavioral research involving human subjects [and] develop guidelines which should be followed in such research to assure that it is conducted in accordance with such principles" (Federal Register, 1975, 51638). From the work of this interdisciplinary committee emerged ethical principles that have been the basis of federal regulation of biomedical research.

Federal regulations with implications for research are continually being promulgated, reviewed, updated, and revised. These regulations can be found through indexes to the Code of Federal Regulations and the Federal Register. They govern the conduct of any studies receiving federal funds as well as research conducted at institutions supported by federal monies.

ETHICAL CODES

At least 33 different sets of formalized guidelines for the ethical conduct of research have been developed since World War II. They all seem to reflect five basic principles (Davis and Krueger, 1980, p. 5).

1. A research subject is a person who volunteered to participate in the research on the basis of having all the necessary information so that his decision will be a truly informed one.
2. The research subject should be allowed to withdraw from the study at any point if and when he wishes to do so.
3. All necessary risks should be eliminated in the research design, and, if appropriate, the research design should have been tried out with prior animal studies.
4. The benefits of the study, either to society or to the individual or preferably to both, should outweigh the risks to the subject involved.

5. The experimentation should be conducted only by individuals qualified to do so.

Following are summaries of some of the codes and regulations that have had significant impact upon the ethical conduct of medical and nursing research. It is important to remember that final accountability and responsibility for the ethical and legal conduct of a project always resides ultimately with the investigator. Laws and codes provide a foundation on which societal norms of conduct are established, but morality (ethics) cannot be legislated and controlled completely by laws.

Nuremburg Code of 1947. The first written set of principles to guide ethical action in research was the Nuremburg Code of 1947. From the famous Nuremburg trials emerged the first set of standards for judging physicians and scientists conducting biomedical experiments. The predominant principle evolving from this code was the principle of informed and voluntary consent. This code subsequently became a prototype for other codes relating to human subjects.

Declaration of Helsinki of 1961. This set of principles, developed by the World Medical Association, reinforced the ideas contained in the Nuremburg Code. The Declaration of Helsinki also addressed the problems arising when clinical research is carried out within the context of professional care.

Professional Codes of Ethics. Most professional groups also have their own codes of research ethics (for instance, the American Medical Association and the American Psychological Association). Within nursing, ethical conduct in research is guided by at least two sets of standards. They are: *The Code for Nurses with Interpretive Statements* (1976) and *Human Rights Guidelines for Nurses in Clinical and Other Research* (1975) [Appendix A]. The Canadian Nurses' Association has also adopted a code of nursing research ethics.

PROTECTING HUMAN SUBJECTS

Informed Consent

Informed consent means the knowing consent of an individual (or his legally authorized representative) who is so situated as to be able to exercise free power or choice without undue inducement or any element of force, fraud, deceit, duress, or other form of constraint or coercion. Eight basic elements are specified to constitute informed consent (Table 14–1) (*Federal Register*, Vol. 46, No. 17, Janurary 27, 1981, Paragraph 50.25[a], [1]–[8]). They are:

1. *A statement that the study involves research, an explanation of the purposes of the research and the expected duration of the subject's participation, a description of the procedures to be followed, and identification of any procedures which are experimental.* This is accomplished by providing the subject with a written information sheet (usually separate from the consent). This information sheet explains in everyday language what will be done in the conduct of the study. Since research is sometimes not clearly

Table 14–1. BASIC ELEMENTS OF INFORMED CONSENT

1. A statement that the study involves research, an explanation of the purposes of the research and the expected duration of the subject's participation, a description of the procedures to be followed, and identification of any procedures which are experimental.
2. A description of any reasonably foreseeable risks or discomforts to the subject.
3. A description of any benefits to the subject or to others which may reasonably be expected from the research.
4. A disclosure of appropriate alternative procedures or courses of treatment, if any, that might be advantageous to the subject.
5. A statement describing the extent, if any, to which confidentiality of records identifying the subject will be maintained and that notes the possibility that the Food and Drug Administration may inspect the records if investigational drugs or devices are involved.
6. For research involving more than minimal risk, an explanation as to whether any compensation and an explanation as to whether any medical treatments are available if injury occurs and, if so, what they consist of or where further information may be obtained.
7. An explanation of whom to contact for answers to pertinent questions about the research and research subjects' rights, and whom to contact in the event of a research-related injury to the subject.
8. A statement that participation is voluntary, that refusal to participate will involve no penalty or loss of benefits to which the subject is otherwise entitled.

distinguishable from treatment, the fact that it is a study must be clearly stated. Some institutions require a statement such as "You are being asked to participate in a research study."

2. *A description of any reasonably foreseeable risks or discomforts to the subject.* Physical risks are those that have the potential for causing harm through altering the physical condition of a subject. Psychosocial risks may be more difficult to identify since these may appear very differently to the researcher and the research participant. A pilot study may be a valuable means by which the relative pain or anxiety provoked by a particular protocol can be estimated. Another suggestion to avoid the question of risk—especially psychological stress—is to seek out situations for study where the phenomenon occurs naturally.
3. *A description of any benefits to the subject or to others which may reasonably be expected from the research.* This is an element that is sometimes neglected by beginning researchers. In the concern over disclosing potential risks, one often forgets to mention the positive benefits that might accrue. Keep in mind that all benefits—both to the individual subject and also to patients at large—should be mentioned. Otherwise, subjects have no basis upon which to weigh their own risk-benefit ratio.
4. *A disclosure of appropriate alternative procedures or courses of treatment, if any, that might be advantageous to the subject.* This stipulation is relevant to therapeutic research. The patient has the right to know what other treatment choices are available.
5. *A statement describing the extent, if any, to which confidentiality of records identifying the subject will be maintained and that notes the possibility that the Food and Drug Adminstration may inspect the records if investigational drugs or devices are involved.* Confidentiality and anonymity of research data are key issues. Although anonymity (when the researcher is unable to link the participant with the data) is often impossible to maintain in clinical studies, subjects must be assured that their privacy will be protected. The researcher needs to assure volunteers that data will be confidential; that is, names or other identifying information will not be communicated with the results of the study.
6. *For research involving more than minimal risk, an explanation as to whether any compensation and an explanation as to whether any medical treatments are available if injury occurs and, if so, what they consist of or where further information may be obtained.*

7. *An explanation of whom to contact for answers to pertinent questions about the research and research subjects' rights, and whom to contact in the event of a research-related injury to the subject.*
8. *A statement that participation is voluntary, that refusal to participate will involve no penalty or loss of benefits to which the subject is otherwise entitled.* Prospective subjects must be assured that they can refuse to participate or withdraw from a study at any time without jeopardizing any future treatment or care.

Questions Often Asked About Consent

- Is consent required for a chart review? Sometimes. The institutional review committee is best able to determine if the use of such materials warrants individual consent.
- Is consent necessary when the researcher is making observations of a group in a field setting? In a public setting such as a cafeteria, bus, or street corner, explanations prior to data collection are not usually necessary unless the subjects are to be interviewed. However, if observations take place in a circumscribed setting, such as a waiting room, an explanation and consent should be obtained from someone responsible for the area.
- Is consent required for a control group? Yes. Even though no special treatment or participation will be required of control group members, consent is required because comparative data will be collected and analyzed.
- How informed is informed? Sometimes a researcher does not want to reveal all the facts of a study to avoid biasing results. For example, if the purpose of a study is to determine if structured teaching reduces the need for narcotics after surgery, telling subjects what you are going to measure may make them change their requests for pain shots. In this case, it is acceptable to explain the study in broader terms such as, "We want to determine the effects of different types of teaching on patients who are recovering from surgery." After the study is completed, subjects could then be told the specific variables under study.
- Can consent be informed if deception is involved? The use of deception in research is controversial. When deception is being considered, several questions should be posed: Is the research very

important? If so, is there *no* other way to obtain the data without deception? Would the participants be expected to find it reasonable and to suffer no consequences? Can the subject withdraw at any time? Is there a plan to "debrief" subjects afterward for the purpose of finding and alleviating any stressful aftereffects? If there are satisfactory answers to these questions, then many researchers would concur that deception may sometimes be necessary and ethically acceptable.

Risk-Benefit Ratio

Federal and ethical guidelines dictate that the benefits to the individual subject, to a group, and/or to society as a whole from all research must outweigh the risks of participation. Nursing research, as contrasted with biomedical and pharmacological research, claims few physical risks to subjects. In fact, no known case of physical injury as a direct result of nursing research has ever been reported.

However, the issues of psychological and social stress are extremely difficult to weigh in the risk-benefit ratio. An extreme example of psychological harm to subjects can be found in the now-famous Milgram studies. In this series of studies, subjects were instructed to apply painful electric currents to people who they did not know were actors and who responded as though they were actually receiving the shocks. The aftermath of these experiments was severe psychological trauma to many of the subjects.

Nursing research can potentially carry risks, especially those similar to hazards of other social science investigations, namely, the loss of trust, the discrediting of the profession, and the generation of anxiety and ill will among the populations served.

Research Within the Context of the Helping Relationship

Nurses, physicians, and other helping professionals face a particularly perplexing dilemma when conducting research within the context of their practice with clients with whom they have formed a trusting relationship. Because there is a fundamental trust in the professional, if this trust is violated the effect may be even more adverse than physical pain or psychological stress.

Many people are still not accustomed to the idea that nurses engage in research. When nurses approach subjects to participate in a study, patients are generally willing to get involved, either because nursing research usually appears to be low risk, or possibly because subjects do not realize that the nurse is in a research role. The role of nurse as researcher is not easily comprehensible to many subjects. Thus it is important that the nurse researcher make every effort to emphasize her researcher status.

Types of Research Review

Review committees of peers give an additional element of protection to all participants: subjects, investigator, sponsoring agency, and those responsible for the subjects's welfare in the research. However, not all reviews are conducted with the same purposes in mind. Beginning researchers often confuse the purposes of the different types of review. The purposes of various research review groups are summarized in the following paragraphs.

Institutional Review Boards. Institutional review panels, sometimes called IRB's, Human Subjects Committees, or Human Investigation Committees, are required to govern all research involving human subjects that is supported by the federal government or research conducted at institutions that receive federal support. The intent of these panels is to promote self-regulation by individual research communities.

The review process varies from institution to institution. Generally, the panels are multidisciplinary, are reflective of the research community in the institution, and are charged with three major activities:

1. They must be assured that subjects will not be exposed to physical, psychological, or social injury as a consequence of participating as a research subject.
2. They must ensure that the methods for obtaining subject consent are appropriate with clear, thorough explanations.

3. They must weigh the risk-benefit ratio of a project, ensuring that any potential risks to subjects are clearly outweighed by projected benefits.

Institutional review boards are not specifically charged with critiquing design; their main purpose is to consider ethical matters.

Administrative Clearance. An investigator is always obligated to obtain permission for access to subjects for research from the person or group responsible for the subjects, regardless of whether approval for the project is granted by the institutional review board. Clearance for permission to conduct research on a unit or within a department requires a review of the proposal, the methods, and any inconveniences or interruption to the ongoing activities of the group, and assurances as to how the study will be conducted and communicated.

Funding Agency Review. A funding agency or group reviews a study for the purpose of determining its worthiness for receiving financial support. Factors likely to be of interest to these review panels include: appropriateness to the targeted programs of the funding agency, the significance of the study, strength of the methodology, and assurance that appropriate resources can be made available to ensure the success of the project.

Journal Review. Review of research by the editiorial board of a journal is for the purpose of determining whether or not to publish the project. Factors considered in this review may include: the significance of the problem, the rigor of the methods, the soundness of the conclusions, the logic and clarity of the report, and the potential for overall interest to the subscribers of the journal.

In summary, each form of research review serves a different purpose. Institutional review boards (IRB's) are primarily concerned with the protection of human rights. Administrative reviews are conducted to consider the practicalities of allowing institutional access to a given set of patients or subjects. Review for purposes of funding is to determine the rigor and scientific merit of a project in order to make a judgment to justify the allocation of resources for a particular project. Journal review of a study considers quality and also potential interest to the publication's readership.

It is evident that some of these functions will necessarily overlap. For example, an IRB cannot weigh the risk-benefit ratio of a project without also evaluating to some degree the rigor of the methods. Similarly, those conducting administrative and funding reviews would certainly want to be assured of protection of human rights. These distinct but subtle differences are often confused.

Populations at Risk

A number of abhorrant examples of flagrant violations of human rights in vulnerable populations has led to concern over the rights of these groups. One of the more well-known instances occurred in the 1960's at the Jewish Chronic Disease Center in Brooklyn, New York, where researchers injected live cancer cells beneath the skin of nonconsenting geriatric patients. As late as the early 1970's, reports surfaced concerning a study on the long-term effects of syphilis in which researchers withheld treatment from a number of black men in Tuskegee, Alabama in order to determine the natural history of their disease.

Populations at risk, or vulnerable populations, are considered to be those people with decreased opportunity to exercise informed consent. The following section describes some of the groups usually considered to be at risk and guidelines for research with such groups.

Elderly and Dying Patients. Aging and terminal illness, though strikingly different in many ways, are considered together because the ethical issues surrounding each are similar. In many respects, dying patients share the plight of the elderly in that their physical, mental, social, and psychological conditions may reduce their competence and freedom and thus make them particularly vulnerable to exploitation. It would seem logical that many of the same protective guidelines proposed for the aged might also be needed for dying patients.

One of the ethical issues concerns the frame of reference in which the subject gives consent. The elderly or dying patient grasps for immortality. At life's end there is a strong desire to leave one's mark on the world and to make some societal contribution. This may be particularly acute if the individual feels that his life to that point has had little meaning. Caught at this particularly vulnerable time, the subject demonstrates increased altruism and a need to be needed, and may tend to consent to research that he might not otherwise permit.

Additionally, the deteriorating physical and mental condition often present in dying or elderly patients has the potential to hinder competence and ability to reason.

An added factor is the fact that no one can accurately predict that a patient will indeed die within a specified time frame. The psychological influences on the will to live and the will to die are well known. It may be that labeling a person as "dying" may in inself hasten the death of that person.

Terminally ill patients pose unique situations for researchers because of a number of reasons. First, when patients are too closely scrutinized during the sensitive and private dying period, the question arises as to whether or not this violates the usual standards for privacy and dignity. The nurse researcher must also remember that the dying patient may not be the only subject involved. Family members with close ties to the dying person may be equally vulnerable to risk, as it may be cruel and damaging for a family member to observe experimentation on a loved one.

Warren T. Reich (1978, p. 331) describes three safeguards for elderly subjects that could easily apply to dying subjects as well. They are:

1. The review process should include the perspective of elderly [dying] persons who are not institutionally committed to the research.
2. Some special assessment of the competence of the elderly [dying] may be required, if this can be done without undue offense against the principle of respect for persons.
3. The additional judgment of a third party such as a relative or a patient advocate . . . may assist in providing the necessary assurance of competence and freedom.

Prisoners. Prisoners have been considered less able to exercise informed consent owing to a number of reasons. First, inmates are incarcerated, usually against their will, and have been forcefully removed from their homes, families, and friends; they have lost many of their civil rights, as well as having been subjected to all the degradations and deprivations of imprisonment. Inmates may perceive coercion by the mere fact that investigators have been allowed in the prison and have access to the captive population. Another factor is that living conditions may be so wretched that they could influence a prisoner's decision to participate in order to be released from these conditions for a short time, even if the experiment poses some risk.

Since prison social systems are confined and closed, researchers must also be very careful in publishing or sharing results, taking care that inmates are not able to identify each other, which would destroy anonymity.

In some respects, students, or any captive group for that matter, can be considered similar to prisoners and may potentially be vulnerable to the same risks.

Children and the Mentally Retarded. These groups are considered together because of the similar concerns that their immature or dependent status raises. Because they are relatively helpless or powerless, they are open to abuse of various types. A classic example of exploitation of mentally retarded persons occurred in Willowbrook, New York, where hepatitis experiments were conducted that were clearly non-therapeutic and posed a high risk for the subjects.

In the case of children and the retarded, trends point in the direction that these groups are being regarded as persons and should be awarded their due rights as are other people. In order to maximize their rights, researchers should obtain consent from any child who is capable at seven years (or older, if retarded). In addition, researchers also need to obtain permission from the parents or guardian in a manner that maximizes their understanding of the research.

A few exceptions regarding parental permission are usually recognized. They include:

1. Research related to adolescents involving treatment they legally may receive without parental consent.
2. Research that involves minimal risk and mature minors.
3. Research designed to understand and meet the needs of abused and neglected children.
4. Research involving children whose parents are legally or functionally incompetent.
5. Emancipated minors.

Fetuses. One of the incidents that triggered concern about the use of human fetuses in research occurred when American scientists were purportedly utilizing American funds in Scandinavia for a research project requiring decapitation of fetuses and the use of their heads for experimental purposes. The controversy that continues is whether or not the fetus is, in fact, a person and, as such, has rights. Although the Supreme Court has ruled that a fetus is not a person until it is able to be maintained separate from its mother, states differ in their interpretation and their protection of rights of fetuses.

In summary, any society can be judged by the way it treats its most vulnerable individuals. Using minors and groups with limited civil freedom as research subjects can be justified, in most instances, only if there are benefits that will accrue in the future to them or to others in similar situations or classes.

ETHICAL DILEMMAS

The boundaries between research and the accepted practice of medicine or other professional practice are not always clear and distinct. It is generally accepted that research involves activities that have as their main purpose the immediate goal of furthering knowledge rather than meeting patients' needs. In clinical research, practitioner-investigators have dual responsibilities for patient care and for research to advance the scientific base of the profession. When these two domains overlap, as they often do in clinical research, then ethical dilemmas surface.

One dilemma relates to the conflict that may arise within the patient who also serves dual roles as both patient and subject. Lay people often do not discriminate between research and therapy. Especially if the patient perceives his case to be "hopeless," he may cling to any "last-ditch" effort in the hope that it might help him as an individual.

Accessibility of patients for nursing research projects may sometimes become a sticky issue. In some institutions nurse researchers must still secure physicians' permission to use patients for nursing research. Physicians, who often do not understand the merit of nonexperimental and social science methods, are sometimes reluctant to "let" their patients participate. As a result, ethical and moral questions can be raised concerning a patient's "right" to participate in a project if he so chooses. (Of course, communication with the intent of informing all professionals involved with a patient in a research study is common courtesy.)

Often nurses are expected to participate in research protocols as a condition of employment or they may be data collectors within research projects conducted by others. When nurses do participate in the research of others, it may be possible to negotiate with the principal investigators for joint authorship or to use the information obtained to write a report of the nursing implications of the study.

Informed consent applies to these situations as well; the nurses who participate in a study must be told of this expectation prior to employment. Furthermore, nurses need to be informed of the manifestations of any potentially harmful effects to patients under their care and should have the means available for alleviating them.

Although meticulous attention to the ethics of research is a professional mandate and responsibility, some would argue that the pendulum on ethical concerns has swung too far toward the side of caution. There is some sentiment that we have become so preoccupied with the dangers and potential ethical violations of research that we may have discouraged valuable investigative efforts (Robb, 1982). There is no doubt that this and other related issues will be a source for debate in the coming years.

ELEMENTS FOR CRITIQUE OF HUMAN RIGHTS PROTECTION

- Has the risk-benefit ratio been considered?
- Are the procedures ethical?
- Is informed consent obtained?
- Are provisions made to protect populations at risk?
- Are privacy and anonymity safeguarded?
- Are subjects free to withdraw from the study at any time?
- Is there evidence that the study was approved by appropriate review boards?
- Are efforts made to minimize risks to subjects?
- Is there evidence that the researcher has made provisions for needed care and treatment when appropriate?

Questions and Activities

1. *Describe the components of informed consent.*
2. *Discuss the dilemmas involved when research is conducted within the context of the helping relationship.*
3. *If you were a member of an institutional review board, how would you assess the risk-benefit ratio of a specific study?*
4. *What are the particular ethical problems involved in research with the following groups?*
   a. *Children*
   b. *Prisoners*
   c. *Elderly*
   d. *Fetuses*
   e. *Mentally retarded*
   f. *Animals*
5. *How has the concern for the protection of human subjects influenced the kinds of studies currently being undertaken?*

Bibliography

American Hospital Association (1970). *Patient's bill of rights*. Chicago: American Hospital Association.

American Nurses' Association (1985). *Human rights guidelines for nurses in clinical and other research*. Kansas City, MO: American Nurses' Association.

Armiger, B. (1977). Ethics of nursing research: Profile, principles, perspective. *Nursing Research, 26*(5), 330–336.

Curtin, L., and Flaherty, M. J. (1982). *Nursing ethics: Theories and pragmatics*. Bowie, MD: Robert J. Brady.

Davis, A. J. (1984). Ethical issues in nursing research. *Western Journal of Nursing Research, 6*(2), 251–252.

Davis, A. J., and Krueger, J. C. (1980). *Patients, nurses, and ethics*. New York: American Journal of Nursing Co.

Lewis, M. (1981). Comments on some ethical, legal, and clinical issues affecting consent in treatment, organ transplants, and research in children. *Journal of the American Academy of Child Psychology, 20*(3), 581–596.

Oberst, M. T. (1979). Research ethics. Part 1: Randomized clinical trials. *Cancer Nursing, 2*, 385–386.

Reich, W. T. (1978). Ethical issues related to research involving elderly subjects. *The Gerontologist, 18*, 326–337.

Robb, S. S. (1982). The Elderly in LTC: Protected to death from research? *Reflections, 8*, 7.

Robb, S. S. (1983). Beware the "informed consent." *Nursing Research, 32*, 132.

Robb, S. S., and Kelly, M. S. (1984). The use and abuse of volunteers in research. *Reflections, 10*, 12.

Scott, D. W. (1982). Ethical issues in nursing research: Access to human subjects. *Topics in Clinical Nursing, 4*(1), 74–83.

World Medical Association (1964). *Declaration of Helsinki: Recommendations guiding doctors in clinical research*. New York: World Medical Association.

15

Facilitating Clinical Projects

OBJECTIVES

After completing this chapter the reader will be able to:

1. Discuss factors within the clinical setting that may present obstacles to the researcher.
2. List the advantages and disadvantages to collaboration with colleagues.
3. Apply time management techniques to the research situation
4. Describe the process of consultation in a research context.
5. Discuss factors to consider in negotiating a clinical site.
6. Suggest strategies for garnering financial and political research support.
7. Describe how change can be managed in the conduct of clinical projects.

Knowledge of the research process alone cannot guarantee a successful project. There are far too many examples of brilliantly designed projects that never made it off the ground because the researcher did not have the capacity to overcome the formidable hurdles that face a clinical investigator. Some of these hurdles relate to factors within the investigator, such as lack of motivation, time constraints, or deficient skills, while other hurdles relate to available resources, human, financial, and otherwise. This chapter will address some of the real-world problems that confront the clinical researcher and will offer suggested alternatives to overcoming them.

CHALLENGES WITHIN THE REAL WORLD OF CLINICAL RESEARCH

Conducting research in the clinical arena presents challenges unknown to the laboratory researcher. While the process is certainly similar for clinical and bench researchers, and many of the obstacles are familiar to both, research with humans in the clinical setting presents a number of problems that challenge the novice and experienced researcher alike. Several characteristics within the clinical setting may lead to frustration.

Low Degree of Predictability. Because clinical research deals with human beings within social systems, all of the random behaviors and idiosyncrasies inherent within them will be potential problems for the researcher. People do not respond to diseases on schedule and clinical phenomena do not announce their occurrence.

Limitless Confounding Variables. The number of potential intervening factors in a clinical study is practically limitless. Patient factors (such as perception, sensitivities, coping mechanisms), situational factors (such as family support, group dynamics), personnel factors (such as staffing levels, educational preparation, motivation), environmental factors (such as temperature, noise), and systemic factors (such as economics, legal and social forces and trends) all can act solely or in combination to confound the research question under study.

Scarcity of Subjects. Researchers have an "inside joke" that says if you want to eliminate a certain clinical problem, all you have to do is start to study it and, miraculously, it disappears. Graduate students, in particular, seem to be susceptible to the phenomenon that whenever one starts to study a group, it immediately becomes scarce. It must be a corollary to Murphy's law that subjects with a particular characteristic are in inverse proportion to the degree to which they are being studied.

One way to at least estimate whether availability of subjects is a potential problem is to investigate the problem prior to the study. Check with the medical records department to see how many patients with a particular characteristic were admitted in previous years. Check clinic records to see how many patients keep return appointments. Conduct a pilot test. Another potential method for circumventing this dilemma is to use single-subject designs as described in Chapter 6.

COLLABORATION WITH COLLEAGUES

Completing a research project, as with any major undertaking, can often seem to be an overwhelming task. Motivation, interest, and energy must remain high to keep momentum going. Many worthwhile projects are relegated to back drawers when these factors wane.

One suggestion, particularly for novice researchers, is to combine efforts with a colleague who shares a similar interest. Or better yet, link up with an experienced researcher who is willing to enter into a mentor relationship.

These types of liaisons present several advantages over "going it alone." As the old saying goes, "Two heads are often better than one." No one is expert (or particularly interested for that matter) in all aspects of the research process. The most complementary relationship is one in which two people can enhance each other's strong areas, for example a strong content person with a strong methodology person.

Secondly, collaboration can be beneficial in terms of motivation. When one partner is down, most often the other is up and can provide that necessary spark to proceed. It is also a factor in sticking to deadlines, since one is less likely to hold up a colleague's progress but it is very easy to let research be a low priority when there is only oneself to feel the consequences.

One caution is necessary when discussing the idea of collaboration. Competition and territoriality are potential hazards if ground rules are not clearly established from the outset. Good intentions, good will, and friendship are not enough to prevent these potential problems in even the most solid professional relationships. Questions that should be addressed very early on (at least in general terms) include division of responsibilities, lines of accountability and authority, and questions of credit and authorship on completed work. These issues are much easier to resolve at the outset when they can be addressed in theoretical terms than they are in the midst of a disagreement or dilemma.

MULTIDISCIPLINARY RESEARCH

A variant on the theme of collaboration is the idea of multidisciplinary research. This situation is becoming much more common in nursing and health care and offers a number of advantages. The richness that can be added to a project when a problem is seen from several unique professional perspectives is a major asset. In addition, each discipline usually can contribute different resources to the project; for example, a basic scientist may have laboratory skills and equipment, whereas a nurse researcher has more access to the clinical population.

The cautions about laying ground rules at the onset (discussed in the previous section) are also applicable here, perhaps more so since different professional groups may have different established norms.

FINDING TIME

One of the most frequently heard laments from nurses is, "I don't have the time to do research." While it is true that nurses usually have extremely demanding jobs and numerous important responsibilities, the truth of the matter is that we can all find time to do the things that we value. Through the conscientious application of time management techniques, the nurse researcher can learn to work "smarter" and thus tackle the time demon.

One reason that nurses perceive there is no time to do research is that they look at the process as one enormous overwhelming project that is a single entity. They fail to realize, however, that it is merely the sum of a large number of small, easily managed subtasks. For example, some people may be so intimidated by the idea of conducting a literature review that they would not know where to begin. However, if viewed as merely a series of substeps—listing key topic areas, requesting a computerized search, identifying entry points, retrieving and reviewing articles, and summarizing articles—then the process becomes less formidable.

Setting goals is a key activity in managing time on a research project. Without a roadmap of where to go, it is less likely that one will arrive. The steps of the research process can be used as a guide in setting major goals, which are then broken down into subgoals.

Once goals are established, one can develop a specific weekly schedule by attaching times and dates to each goal and subgoal. This process is not unlike budgeting—in fact, it is a budgeting of time. By setting down an estimated time schedule and then evaluating progress against the actual schedule, it is like comparing actual expenditures, in this case time instead of money, with what was previously planned. It is important that the deadlines be reasonable and realistic, remembering that things generally take longer than anticipated. When unrealistic time estimates are imposed, this will serve only to increase stress. Build in "catch-up time" each week for completing tasks not finished when originally scheduled. If this time is not needed, it could be used to get a head start on the next week's scheduled tasks. An example of a projected timetable for a small clinical project is shown in Table 15–1.

Some researchers find it helpful to create lists of things to be done. For example, make a list each week of the major and minor things to be accomplished and rank them in priority order. In this way, when time is available, the researcher can look at the list and decide what could reasonably be accomplished within that time period. For example, if only five minutes are available, a phone call could be accomplished, whereas another activity might take a longer period of time. One danger, of course, is that the quick and easier tasks may get completed first with the larger, more difficult tasks remaining uncompleted at the end of the week. Thus, it is a good idea to schedule blocks of time and to use these blocks for the more challenging segments of the project. Tackling the less desirable jobs first is also a good rule.

Table 15–1. EXAMPLE OF A FLOW CHART

Request on-line bibliographic search	Week 1
Review literature	Weeks 2—6
Develop problem statement and hypotheses	Weeks 3–5
Design methodology	Weeks 4—8
Locate research instrument	Weeks 7–9
Request administrative and IRB approvals	Weeks 9—12
Train interviewers	Weeks 9—12
Pilot test research instrument	Weeks 10—12
Negotiate for access to clinical population	Week 12
Data collection	Weeks 12—20
Coding of data forms and data entry	Weeks 20—25
Data analysis	Weeks 26—30
Write final report	Weeks 31—34

USING CONSULTANTS

Even the most experienced researchers recognize the necessity and value of using consultants in conducting research. Advice from experts can often make the difference between an average project and one that is outstanding.

However, sometimes nurse researchers are reluctant to use consultants. They may be embarrassed about asking for help, mistakenly believing that they should be able to do the entire project independently. Or, they may imagine that they will be embarrassed and feel inadequate or stupid. They may also fear that they would not know the right questions to ask or that the consultant may end up "taking over" the project.

Such fears are unfounded if the nurse researcher understands the nature of the consultation process and knows how to use a research consultant properly. Suggestions for working with consultants are summarized in Table 15–2. Most importantly, one should remember that the consultation is a service or a conference between professionals.

Finding consultants is not always easy, depending upon the area of need. One area in which consultation is frequently necessary is statistical analysis. Asking people who have previously done research can sometimes help you identify statistical consultants. They are sometimes found in the data centers of universities and hospitals, or in mathemetics or epidemiology departments. Clinical consultants are usually easier for nurses to identify, since nurses often are exposed to them in the course of clinical work.

One should not be limited to one's own institution in locating consultants. They may be found in local universities. In addition, community organizations, such as the Heart Association or the Lung Association, usually have research committees whose members are often willing to consult with other researchers. Also, remember that national experts are available by phone; often major researchers are very eager to provide assistance to other researchers interested in similar problems.

Table 15–2. GUIDELINES FOR USING RESEARCH CONSULTANTS

Be considerate of the consultant's time and punctual for meetings.
Do your homework before meeting with the consultant. The consultant will need to have background information including hypotheses, data forms, and protocols.
Set clear expectations about the nature of help that is requested. A consultant is not a mindreader.
Clearly define the parameters of the relationship. Remember, it is *your* study and you are in the best position to assess the overall needs and directions. A consultant is there only to provide suggestions.
Try not to hold tightly to preconceived ideas about what you think needs to be done. Flexibility and an open mind are essential.
Be candid. If data collection did not go exactly as planned, don't try to hide or sidestep limitations. A consultant is not there to be judgmental and may be able to help you remedy some flaws.
Don't expect the consultant to solve all your problems. A consultant cannot perform miracles on a poorly conceived or poorly executed study.
Don't expect the consultant to do all of the work for you. For instance, if you use a statistician for data analysis, don't assume that she will also do the computer programming.
Expect to pay the consultant for her services. Negotiate the cost at the outset.

The initial contact with a consultant is crucial. It is during this period that the nurse researcher outlines the nature of the request. Both parties should clearly understand the nature of the problem, know what is expected of each party involved, and agree on a tentative time schedule.

Throughout the process, be prepared to work *with* the consultant. If a particular problem is merely "handed over" to a consultant to solve, then a different type of relationship exists and different ground rules may apply. One gets best advantage of the consultant when each person contributes toward problem resolution, rather than expecting unilateral service. For example, the researcher should come to the statistician prepared with clear hypotheses and as much descriptive information about the data as possible. An outgrowth of mutual participation is usually that the researcher also gains new knowledge in the process, and the result may be that the next time a similar situation is encountered, it can be handled independently.

Researchers often forget that they have a choice of accepting or rejecting a consultant's advice. Most often the recommendations are reasonable, but only the investigator knows best the overall picture of the project and is in the best position to judge the merit of the advice. For example, a consultant may be very knowledgeable about statistics but may know very little about the clinical problem being researched. Remember that the consultant is an *invited colleague* and that the most satisfying results are achieved when you both work together as professionals.

FINDING A CLINICAL SITE

Not all nurse researchers are fortunate to be able to conduct research within their own clinical practice area. It may be that they do not have a clinical practice, that they cannot gain appropriate approvals, or that the setting does not meet criteria for the study. In these circumstances, the researcher must find a setting where she can conduct her research. Hodgman (1978) suggests several questions that should be asked concerning clinical agencies:

1. Can the clinical agency provide the data?
2. Are the projected data collection dates reasonable?
3. Will the study interfere with ongoing or projected research within the agency?

4. Does the study duplicate current or projected research within the agency?
5. Does any aspect of the study conflict with institutional or departmental philosophy, objectives, or policy?
6. Must the study be approved by the institutional review boards?

Negotiating for access to a clinical site should usually begin with the middle management level, such as an associate director, because these are the people within an organization who usually have authority and responsibility to move up and down the institutional hierarchy. It helps to give references about your own qualifications and to note official sponsorship from your own setting, if possible. These will give credibility to your request. Also, be prepared to share specific details of the study and have data collection instruments and protocols available. Anticipate that you will need to participate in several meetings with both the administration and the staff in order to explain your project. Of course, the agency providing the setting will want to be assured that your study meets ethical criteria and may require you to submit the study to their institutional review board as well as your own.

GARNERING SUPPORT

Financial Support

Conducting research does not need to be needlessly expensive. Estimating expenses for a project is not always easy. Some researchers who do not intend to request funding may think that they do not need to prepare a budget, but projecting expenses will help to ensure that there are sufficient resources to undertake the project. Sometimes one might think a project is not expensive, but getting everything on paper proves otherwise. Things do add up. It is better to know this beforehand rather than run the risk that a good project would have to be scrapped midstream because of a lack of financial support.

A basic budget should include estimated costs for:

1. Library computer searches.
2. Data collection instruments (costs for developing or costs for purchasing).
3. Obtaining equipment and supplies.

4. Salaries for data collectors.
5. Clerical services for typing and duplicating.
6. Postage and/or phone calls.
7. Consultant fees.
8. Computer time.

Many times researchers can use imaginative ways to minimize expenses on a project. Some examples would be using students or other volunteers who might be interested in the project, borrowing equipment from laboratories or other researchers, or asking for donations of supplies from drug companies or other groups. By use of these and other measures, many projects can be conducted at minimal expense.

However, some projects, because of their nature, will require some financial resources to complete. In such cases, various avenues are open and appropriate for funding of nursing research. One thing is certain; you will not get financial support unless you ask for it. Even in economic hard times, some available research money goes unawarded owing to lack of applications.

Sources of Funds

Institutional Sources. Many hospitals, universities, and schools of nursing have research money that is available, often on a competitive basis, for the support of their own projects. Often these funds are specifically earmarked for beginning researchers, in the hopes that they will provide "seed" money for investigations that have the potential to develop into programs qualifying for external funding. In addition, department heads often have "slush funds" available for the support of ad hoc projects. Another possibility is unit funds, which often result from gifts from patients; these could be potential support for a nursing research project.

Private Sources. Sources of private funds are varied and much more available than many imagine. They can include:

1. Foundations.
2. Industry (drug companies, supply houses).
3. Professional organizations (Sigma Theta Tau, AORN, AACN).
4. Community agencies (American Heart Association, American Cancer Society).

5. Special interest groups (elderly, ostomates).
6. Alumni organizations.
7. Church groups.

Governmental Sources. Many states have departments and commissions that fund health-related research. At the federal level, the Department of Health and Human Services (HHS) is the most likely source of research funding. The divisions of the Public Health Service of the department of HHS that are most likely to fund projects for investigators in nursing are:

1. The National Institutes of Health (NIH), which includes the Heart, Lung and Blood Institute, the Institute of Medicine, the Institute on Aging, and others.
2. Alcohol, Drug Abuse, and Mental Health Administration (ADAMHA)
3. Health Resources Administration (HRA), which includes the Division of Nursing.
4. Health Services Administration (HSA).
5. Food and Drug Administration (FDA).
6. Centers for Disease Control (CDC).

For both private and governmental funds, books, catalogs, periodicals, and computer data bases are available to describe criteria and application procedures. Ask your librarian for assistance in locating these guides. Writing a grant proposal is not within the scope of this book, but a number of good guides are available in most libraries. It is also advisable to seek assistance from an experienced investigator if you are writing a grant proposal. In addition, in many cases consultants are available from the funding agency to assist in the preparation of a grant request.

BUILDING A POLITICAL SUPPORT BASE

Any research project, but particularly a project that occurs within the context of an existing social system, is doomed to failure if it does not have the support of those outside the research situation. No project occurs in a vacuum, and the more complex the system, the more the project is likely to require a political support base.

It is essential to identify the influential members within the setting, both the formal and the informal leaders. For example, formal leaders might be the head nurse and the medical director of a unit. However, if the project involves special handling of patients' charts, for example, then the unit clerk might very well be the more influential person in that situation.

Whoever the leaders are, it is important to ensure that they support you. They should ideally have an investment in the success of your project, for if they do, then they will be instrumental in facilitating its completion. If they do not see the project as valuable (or worse yet, if they see it as a threat), they can do much to sabotage its progress.

Ensuring the support of significant people can be time-consuming but is well worth the effort. Suggestions include using them as initial consultants; asking their advice; keeping them informed; making sure that they understand the positive value of the research, especially any direct advantages that may accrue to them, the system, or their patients; ensuring that you also have the support of their superiors and appropriate institutional approvals; and minimizing intrusion and disruption in their system.

MANAGING CHANGE IN THE CONDUCT OF CLINICAL PROJECTS

The implementation of research in a clinical setting, especially a setting unaccustomed to research, will proceed much more smoothly if the investigator considers the application of principles of change in the process. Clinical research does not occur in isolation, so its implementation must be articulated within the context of the setting in which it occurs. This process generally means some degree of change for the participants.

1. *Anticipate impact on the system.* Change at any level creates complementary changes in related parts of the system. In much the same way, a research project can lead to intended as well as unintended consequences. It is important for the researcher to attempt to anticipate what impact the activity will have.
2. *Involve decision-makers.* The more one can get input from the key people in a situation (that is, those who control resources), the more likely it is that they will feel vested in the outcome. If their

advice is not solicited, the researcher runs the risk of alienating them from the process.

3. *Capitalize on the informal structure.* Official support of a project means little if one does not also have the support of those at the grass roots. It is important to identify members of a group who have informal influence, and win their favor.
4. *Involve the participants.* The most ideal situation occurs when the researcher is an actual member of the staff or group where the research will occur. It is the nature of groups to be suspicious of outsiders, so trust will be increased if the staff views the researcher as "one of us" or at least "on our side" or acting in the staff's best interest.

   If the researcher is an outsider and is attempting to gain support for a project, then a good technique is to involve participants when possible. For example, the staff members can contribute ideas to the design of the project or they can help in writing subsections of the proposal or in outlining protocols, provided that these activities will not jeopardize the internal validity of the project.

   In some projects, it may be possible and desirable to involve staff in actual data collection, either as data collectors or in helping to recruit subjects. Many times staff will welcome this diversity to their day and they will become much more interested in the successful outcome of the project. A caution is needed here to prevent exploitation of staff at the expense of their usual duties.
5. *Anticipate resistance.* In any change venture, a predictable cycle of resistance can be anticipated. Resistance can't be ignored, for it often serves to warn us of real threats in the situation. Thus, it is important to let resisters have their say, but then to mobilize and channel the resistance in a positive way.
6. *Emphasize the positive.* Let the participants know the projected outcomes of the study. Attempt to link the potential benefits of the study to their personal situations.
7. *Pilot test.* Change is easier to handle if it is introduced gradually and tested first to work out the bugs.
8. *Capitalize on initial success.* "Nothing succeeds like success." Let people know how well the project is going. If you are enthusiastic, others will follow.

Questions and Activities

1. *What realities are involved when undertaking a clinical study?*
2. *Discuss the advantages and disadvantages of research collaboration with other colleagues.*
3. *What information should you gather in preparation for using a statistical consultant?*
4. *Suppose you are planning a study to evaluate a sibling visitation program. What sources might you consider for financial support?*
5. *Suppose you are planning to conduct a small study on your unit and you would like to use your fellow staff members as data collectors. How might you utilize the principles of change theory to engage their support and cooperation?*

Bibliography

Campos, R. G. (1980). Acquiring foundation funds. *Journal of Nursing Administration, 10*(6), 16–23.

Hodgman, E. C. (1978). Student research in service agencies. *Nursing Outlook, 26*(9), 558–565.

Jacobson, S. F. (1978). An insider's guide to field research. *Nursing Outlook, 26*(6), 371–374.

Keithley, J. K., Shelley, S., and Benner, J. A. (1979). Help at hand: Using the nurse consultant. *Nursing, 9*(11), 105–112.

Kenneth, H., and Gortner, S. R. (1984). Researchmanship: Some issues in gaining access to subject participants for clinical nursing research. *Western Journal of Nursing Research, 6*(2), 256–258.

Sexton, D. L. (1982). Developing skills in grant writing. *Nursing Outlook, 30*(1), 31–38.

Strombeck, R. D. (1982). The client-consultant relationship: Guidelines for the nursing administrator. *Journal of Nursing Administration, 12*(7–8), 42–46.

White, V. P. (1975). *Grants: How to find out about them and what to do next.* New York: Plenum.

Glossary

Abscissa The horizontal scale (x-axis) of a graph.

Abstract A brief summary of a research study that capsulizes the major points of the methods and findings.

Accidental sample See *Sample.*

Acquiescence response set bias See *Bias.*

Active variable See *Variable.*

Analysis of covariance A statistic combining the basic ideas of analysis of variance and correlational analysis.

Analysis of variance A parametric statistic used to decide whether two or more group variances differ from one another. It is a parametric test.

Anecdotal reports Summaries of events occurring outside of experimental situations that do not generally reflect control of variables. They may take the form of case studies, clinical impressions, observations of situations, or descriptions of programs.

Attribute variable See *Variable.*

Axiom See *Principle.*

Bar chart Depiction of frequencies in bar form, either horizontally or vertically.

Bibliography Citations of materials intended to provide background material or suggestions for further reading.

Bias A process that prejudices, slants, influences, or improperly affects research data.

- **Acquiescence response set bias** A type of scaling bias that reflects subjects' tendency to agree with statements regardless of content.
- **Extreme response set bias** A type of scaling bias in which some people tend to answer with extreme opinions, rather than the middle-of-the-road alternatives.
- **Reactivity bias** A type of bias in which subjects may change their behavior owing to the presence of an observer. Also called reactive measurement effect.

Social desirability bias A type of scaling bias that reflects the tendency of some individuals to misrepresent their attitudes by giving answers that are consistent with prevailing social attitudes.

Biserial correlation A measure of the relationship between a continuous variable and one that is forced into a dichotomy.

Canonical correlation A statistic used to correlate many independent variables with many dependent variables.

Chi square A statistic useful for testing the independence of variables by assessing the discrepancy between observed and expected frequencies. It is non-parametric and is useful for categorical data.

Closed-ended questions Questions for which the investigator provides a set of responses and the respondent chooses the one(s) that most closely match his or her own answers. Also sometimes called closed or fixed alternative format.

Cluster Sample See *Sample.*

Compensatory equalization of treatment See *Internal validity.*

Compensatory rivalry See *Internal validity.*

Compound question See *Double-barreled question.*

Computer-assisted searches Retrieval of bibliographical citations from on-line data bases or compilations of literature within a particular area of interest.

Concept An abstract idea that represents a class or group of things or actions having certain characteristics in common.

Confounding variable See *Intervening variable,* at *Variable.*

Consent See *Informed consent.*

Construct An abstract idea composed of interrelated concepts.

Construct validity See *Validity.*

Content analysis A technique used to make replicable and valid inferences from qualitative data.

Content validity See *Validity.*

Contingency coefficient A statistical value calculated following a chi-square analysis to express the degree of relatedness between two nominal variables.

Continuous variable See *Variable.*

Control group The subjects who are not exposed to the experimental treatment.

Convenience sample See *Sample.*

Correlation The relationship between two or more variables.

Correlational design A study that examines relationships between variables.

Criterion-related validity See *Validity.*

Criterion variable See *Dependent variable,* at *Variable.*

Critical incident report A type of focused observation in which data are recorded only from those specific occurrences that have been found to have a marked significance to the problem under study. Also sometimes called anecdotes.

Cronbach's alpha See *Reliability.*

Cross-sectional study A one-time study of a defined population at a specific time period.

Deduction See *Logical reasoning.*

Degrees of freedom The number of independent observations in a data set.

Demoralization effects See *Internal validity.*

Dependent variable. See *Variable.*

Describing and measuring the dependent variable See *External validity.*

Describing the independent variable See *External validity.*

Descriptive statistics Statistics used to describe, summarize, and characterize sample data.

Diffusion of treatment See *Internal validity.*

Discrete variable See *Variable.*

Discriminant function analysis A statistical technique similar to multiple regression except that the dependent variable is categorical.

Dissertation See *Thesis.*

Double-barreled question A question that implies two separate reponses. Also sometimes called a compound question.

Empirical data Information that can be verified by objective observation or experimentation.

Equal-appearing interval scale See *Thurstone scale,* at *Scale.*

Eta A measure of the relationship between two continuous curvilinear variables.

Event sampling See *Sampling.*

Experimental design A study organized as an experiment, characterized by randomization, manipulation, and control.

Experimental group Subjects who are exposed to the experimental intervention.

Experimentally accessible population versus target population See *External validity.*

Experimenter (Rosenthal) effect See *External validity.*

Exploratory design A design used when there is little information about specific variables.

Ex post facto design A design in which there is no control over an independent variable.

External validity The extent to which findings can be generalized to other people (population validity) and other settings (ecological validity). The following are threats to external validity:

- **Describing and measuring the dependent variable** When the dependent variable is not adequately described, it is impossible to make judgments concerning a study's results.
- **Describing the independent variable** When the experimental procedures are not described, it is impossible to replicate a study.
- **Experimentally accessible population versus target population** When subjects are chosen on the basis of availability, it is not possible to randomly select subjects from a defined population.
- **Experimenter (Rosenthal) effect** When a researcher unknowingly influences subjects' responses.
- **Hawthorne effect** When awareness of being in a study precipitates certain kinds of behavior.
- **Interaction between treatment and subject characteristics** When subject variables such as age and sex interact with a treatment—for example, an exercise intervention—erroneous conclusions may result.
- **Interaction of history and treatment effect** Events occurring when a study is conducted may interfere with the experimental treatment.
- **Interaction of time of measurement and treatment effects** When measurements made before or after the occurrence of a treatment effect fail to capture the effect.
- **Multiple treatment interference** When the results of experimental treatments are confounded by each other.
- **Novelty and disruption effects** When the novelty of the experimental situation supercedes the experimental effects.
- **Pre-test and post-test sensitization** When tests sensitize subjects to expectations (pre-test) or facilitate recall of the experiment (post-test).

Extraneous variable See *Intervening variable*, at *Variable*.

Extreme response set bias See *Bias*.

Factor analysis Statistical method used to explain relationships among many variables in a simplified way.

Field experiment An experiment conducted outside the laboratory in the real world.

Fixed alternative format See *Closed-ended questions*.

Fixed interview See *Standardized interview*, at *Interview*.

Free answer format See *Open-ended questions*.

Frequency distribution A graphic display of raw data.

Frequency polygon A figure constructed from a histogram by placing a dot in the center of each bar and connecting them.

Graph A visual representation of data. Also referred to as a figure or diagram.

Graphic rating scale See *Scale*.

Grounded theory A conceptual framework generated by the use of data.

Hawthorne effect See *External validity*.

Histogram A bar chart representing continuous data in which the bars touch one another.

Historical research A research approach that aims to reconstruct the past to reach conclusions about events or people.

History See *Internal validity*.

Homogeneous Possessing similar characteristics. A homogeneous sample is one in which all members have essential characteristics in common.

Human Subjects Committee/Human Investigations Committee See *Institutional Review Board*.

Hypothesis A statement of relationship between two or more variables.

Independence of observations When the occurrence of one score in no way influences the occurrence of other scores.

Independent variable See *Variable*.

Induction See *Logical reasoning*.

Inferential statistics Statistics used to make inferences to populations using sample data.

Informed consent The knowing permission of an individual or his legally authorized representative, so situated as to be able to exercise free power or choice without undue inducement or any element of force, fraud, deceit, duress, or other form of constraint or coercion.

Institutional Review Board (IRB) A local panel or committee mandated by federal regulations to govern all research involving human subjects that is supported by the federal government or research conducted at institutions that receive federal support. Also called Human Subjects Committees or Human Investigation Committee.

Instrument A tool or measurement device used to collect data.

Instrumentation See *Internal validity*.

Interaction between treatment and subject characteristics See *External validity*.

Interaction of history and treatment effect See *External validity*.

Interaction of time of measurement and treatment effects See *External validity*.

Interaction with selection See *Internal validity*.

Internal validity The extent to which alternative explanations of findings can be eliminated. The following are threats to internal validity:

- **Compensatory equalization of treatment** When control group(s) are subjected to special circumstances and begin to act as the experimental group(s).
- **Compensatory rivalry** When the nature of the experimental intervention is made public, rivalry occurs between the experimental and control groups.
- **Demoralization effects** When differences between the experimental and control groups are amplified because the control group becomes less motivated.
- **Diffusion of treatment** When members of the control group learn about the experimental intervention.
- **History** When an event external to the study design occurs between the pre-test and post-test that influences the results of the post-test.
- **Instrumentation** When precision and accuracy of measuring instruments change between measurements.
- **Interaction with selection** When many factors interact to jeopardize internal validity.
- **Local history** When testing conditions for the experimental and control groups are different.
- **Maturation** When subjects change during an experiment.
- **Mortality** Bias that is the consequence of subjects dropping out.

Selection When there is bias because a random sample was not used.

Statistical regression When a test is readministered, low and high scores have a tendency to regress toward the mean.

Testing When results of a post-test are influenced by the pre-test.

Interval scale See *Scale.*

Intervening variable See *Variable.*

Interview A data collection method employing a verbal questioning technique.

Focused interview Similar to a non-standardized interview in that no specific questions are asked but special attention is given to specific topic areas or ideas.

Interview schedule A series of questions or a guide that is used by the interviewer.

Non-directive interview A type of interview in which the subject has complete freedom to discuss a topic without direction from the interviewer.

Non-standardized interview A type of interview in which the interviewer has freedom to develop each interview in the most appropriate manner for the situation. Also called unstructured or open interview.

Semi-standardized interview A type of interview in which the interviewer may be required to ask a number of specific major questions but she may also be permitted leeway to use alternate questions and/or to probe as she chooses.

Standardized interview A type of interview in which the questions, sequence, and wording are fixed by the investigator. Also called structured or fixed interview.

Isomorphic Means that there is a one-to-one correspondence between two things.

Known-groups technique See *Construct validity.*

Kurtosis Refers to the peakedness of a distribution of numbers.

Laboratory experiment An experiment conducted in a controlled (laboratory) environment.

Law See *Principle.*

Leptokurtic Refers to a tall, skinny distribution of numbers.

Level of significance Designated as alpha or the probability of rejecting a null hypothesis when it is true.

Likert scale See *Scale.*

Local history See *Internal validity.*

Logical reasoning A system of thought that results in forming conclusions, judgments, or inferences.

Deduction A process of reasoning that starts with given premises and attempts to derive valid conclusions. Reasoning from the general abstraction to the particular case.

Induction A process of reasoning that starts with facts about specific situations and attempts to establish general propositions. Reasoning from the particular case to a more general abstraction.

Matching A process whereby subjects are matched in terms of critical variables.

Maturation See *Internal validity.*

Mean The arithmetic average of a distribution of numbers.

Measurement Assigning numbers to properties or attributes of objects according to rules.

Median The midpoint of a distribution of numbers.

Mesokurtic Refers to a normal distribution.

Mode The most frequently occurring number in a distribution of numbers.

Model A simplified, symbolic (sometimes graphic) representation of a theory or conceptual scheme.

Mortality See *Internal validity.*

Multiple correlation A measure of the relationship among at least three variables.

Multiple regression A statistic that describes the relationship between a set of independent variables and a dependent variable.

Multiple-treatment interference See *External validity.*

Multitrait-multimethod See *Construct validity*, at *Validity.*

Negatively skewed When the tail of a distribution is toward low score values.

Nominal scale See *Scale.*

Non-parametric statistics Small-sample, assumption-free statistics.

Non-probability sample See *Sample.*

Non-standardized interview See *Interview.*

Normal curve A bell-shaped curve in which the configuration of values above the middle value is a mirror image of the configuration below the middle.

Novelty and disruption effects See *External validity.*

Null hypothesis A statistical hypothesis claiming no difference between groups.

One-tailed statistical test Type of test used when the alternative (research) hypothesis specifies direction.

Open-ended questions Questions in which the respondent is asked to provide his or her own answer. Also sometimes called free answer format.

Open interview See *Nonstandardized interview*, at *Interview*.

Operational definition A definition of a variable that tells how the variable will be measured.

Ordinal scale See *Scale*.

Ordinate The vertical scale (y-axis) of a graph.

Outcome variable See *Dependent variable*, at *Variable*.

Parallel forms reliability See *Reliability*.

Partial correlation A measure of the relationship between two continuous variables while controlling for the effects of a third.

Pearson product-moment correlation (r) A measure of the relationship between two continuous variables.

Phi coefficient A measure of the relationship between two nominal dichotomous variables.

Pie chart A circle in which the 360 degrees visually represent 100 percent of a sample.

Platykurtic Refers to a flat distribution of numbers.

Point biserial correlation A measure of the relationship between one continuous and one truly dichotomous variable.

Population Any large group of objects or people that can be counted.

Populations at risk Those people or groups with decreased opportunity to exercise informed consent. Also called vulnerable populations.

Positively skewed When the tail of a distribution is toward high score values.

Premise See *Principle*.

Pre-test and post-test sensitization See *External validity*.

Primary data sources Sources in which the data are reported by the person or group that actually gathered the information.

Principle A statement of relationship between two or more concepts. Also called an axiom, law, or premise.

Probability sample See *Sample*.

Prospective study A study conducted to uncover factors associated with a disease or event from the present time forward.

Purposive (judgmental) sample See *Sample.*

Quasi-experimental design A design lacking at least one essential ingredient of an experiment—randomization, manipulation, or control.

Questionnaire A data collection technique consisting of a set of written items requesting a response from subjects; a self-administered interview schedule.

Quota sample See *Sample.*

Random assignment Use of randomization procedures to place members of a sample into experimental and control groups.

Random error Error that is unorderly, without reason.

Range The highest score or value minus the lowest score or value.

Ratio scale A level of measurement that has all of the properties of the interval level plus the property of an absolute zero.

Reactive measurement effect See *Reactivity bias,* at *Bias.*

Reference list Citations of materials intended to document the contents of a written work, limited to those that are actually used in the report.

Reliability Refers to the consistency or stability of measurement. Is a prerequisite for validity.

- **Cronbach's alpha** An approach defined as the average correlation of all possible split-halves of a test.
- **Parallel forms reliability** Two variations of the same instrument are administered to the same group of people and the results correlated.
- **Split-half reliability** A set of items is divided in half and the two halves are correlated.
- **Test-retest reliability** An approach to reliability that compares two administrations of the same measuring instrument.

Research Broadly, any activity whose purpose is to find a valid answer to a question. Specifically, a structured and systematic investigation designed to test a hypothesis and draw conclusions, thereby developing or contributing to generalizable knowledge.

- **Applied research** Investigations undertaken to find solutions to practical problems. Also called practice research.
- **Basic research** Investigations conducted to establish fundamental facts or to develop or test theory. Also called fundamental research.

Nursing research Investigations which develop knowledge about health and the promotion of health over the full life span, care of persons with problems and disabilities, and nursing actions to enhance the ability of individuals to respond effectively to actual or potential health problems. (ANA Commission on Nursing Research, 1981.)

Research design The structure of a study. Is essentially a blueprint.

Research hypothesis A hypothesis used to test existing theory. Each research hypothesis should include only one relationship or difference to be tested.

Research problem That which an investigator intends to study. It is introduced in the beginning of a research report and is similar to a strong legal defense, in that the investigator presents evidence as to why it is a problem.

Research utilization A process directed toward transferring specific research-based knowledge into actual clinical practice.

Response format The structure within which respondents are asked to provide answers to questions, such as filling in blanks, circling words, checking categories.

Retrospective study Examining past events or factors to explain a current event or disease.

Risk-benefit ratio An ethical consideration in which the value of a research study to individual subjects, groups, and/or society as a whole is compared against the potential risks of participation.

Sample A part of a population.

Accidental sample A sample in which no attempt is made to include individuals or elements who meet certain criteria.

Cluster sample A sampling method usually based on geographic location. For example, dividing the U.S. into North, South, East, and West and randomly selecting from each region.

Convenience sample A sample consisting of all subjects who agree to participate.

Non-probability sample A sample in which generalizations cannot be made to the population from which the sample was drawn.

Probability sample A random sample. When a sample is random every member or element of a population has an equal chance of being included.

Purposive (judgmental) sample A sample in which there is an attempt to include individuals or elements who meet certain criteria.

Quota sample Subjects who are available are selected to meet a certain quota, for example, a certain number of staff nurses and a certain number of students.

Simple random sample Sampling that allows every element or member of a population an equal chance of being included.

Stratified random sample An approach that allows random selection from specific parts of a population.

Snowball sample Using initial members of a sample to identify others who might be appropriate study subjects.

Systematic sample A convenient, practical approach in which every other, every third, etc., member in a population is taken into a sample.

Sampling Selection of a part of a population for study.

Event sampling An observational sampling technique in which only events or occurrences of a given class are selected for data collection.

Time sampling An observational sample technique in which a universe of time is identified and a sampling design is employed.

Scale A series of questions in which the responses are graded or weighted in some way to reflect the magnitude or quantity of a variable.

Graphic rating scale A scale in which the variable is qualitatively graded along a continuum and the subject makes a direct rating on the scale.

Interval scale A scale of measurement in which the distance between points on the scale is known.

Likert scale A scale in which items are rated along a continuum that ordinarily contains three to five categories of varying degrees of intensity. Also called a summated rating scale.

Nominal scale A scale in which numbers represent categories.

Ordinal scale A scale in which numbers represent a ranking or ordering.

Semantic differential scale A scale in which the respondent evaluates a concept using a series of bipolar adjectives placed at the endpoints of a seven-point rating scale.

Thurstone scale A battery of statements, each with a specific scale value which denotes the intensity of each statement. Also called the equal appearing interval scale.

Secondary data source A source in which the reporter of the information is not the person or group that actually obtained the data.

Selection See *Internal validity.*

Semantic differential scale See *Scale.*

Simple random sample See *Sample.*

Snowball scale See *Sample.*

Social desirability bias See *Bias.*

Spearman's rho A measure of the relationship between two ordinal variables.

Split-half reliability See *Reliability.*

Standard deviation The square root of the variance.

Standardized interview See *Interview.*

Statistic A numerical value of a variable calculated from sample data.

Statistical estimation Procedure used to estimate population values.

Statistical power The ability of a statistical test to detect significant differences when differences are present.

Statistical regression See *Internal validity.*

Statistical significance When statistical significance is achieved, it is unlikely that a statistical value occurred by just chance alone.

Structured interview See *Standardized interview,* at *Interview.*

Stratified random sample See *Sample.*

Summated rating scale See *Likert scale,* at *Scale.*

Survey research A design for research in which the purpose is to gather information about a large number of people by collecting data from a few.

Systematic error Error that is orderly, that is, error in which all measurements are influenced in the same way. Such an error might be caused by poorly adjusted measuring instruments.

Systematic sample See *Sample.*

t-Test A statistic used to test the difference between two means.

Table A display of data in rows and columns.

Testing See *Internal validity.*

Test-retest reliability See *Reliability.*

Theory An abstract generalization that presents a systematic explanation about the relationships among phenomena. A series of principles, or propositions, regarding the interrelationships among concepts.

Thesis A report of research done by a student in an academic program as a part of a degree requirement. A thesis is generally prepared for a master's degree, while a dissertation is usually written in a doctoral program.

Thurstone scale See *Scale*.

Time sample See *Sample*.

Two-tailed statistical test When the alternate (research) hypothesis does not specify direction.

Type I error The error made in statistical hypothesis testing when a true null hypothesis is rejected.

Type II error The error made in statistical hypothesis testing when a researcher fails to reject a false null hypothesis.

Unstructured interview See *Nonstandardized interview,* at *Interview*.

Validity The extent to which a measuring instrument achieves certain aims. See also *External validity* and *Internal validity*.

Construct validity Validity of the definition of a construct.

Known-groups technique An approach to construct validity in which the idea is to demonstrate that groups inherently different will differ on the construct being measured.

Multitrait-multimethod An approach to construct validation that aims to support a construct by demonstrating that different measures of the same construct will produce similar results while measures of other constructs will produce dissimilar results.

Content validity The extent to which a test reflects the variable it seeks to measure.

Criterion-related validity This approach requires that scores on the test or measuring instrument be related to scores on an external criterion.

Variable Something that has the capacity to vary. A variable can be anything, such as an object, item, factor, or trait.

Active variable A variable to which something is done; that is, the variable is manipulated.

Attribute variable A variable that is observed but not manipulated.

Continuous variable A variable such as blood pressure where there are infinite numbers of values between scores.

Dependent variable A variable that follows and is influenced by another variable, the independent variable. In an experimental situation, changes in a dependent variable are measured following manipulation of an independent variable. Also called a criterion variable or an outcome variable.

Discrete variable A variable composed of separate and discrete categories, such as sex or race.

Independent variable A variable that precedes and possibly affects another variable called the dependent variable.

Intervening variable A variable that may come between an independent variable and a dependent variable and influence or mask changes in the dependent variable. Also called a confounding variable or an extraneous variable.

Variance The average of squared deviations from the mean.

Vulnerable populations See *Populations at risk.*

Appendices

A. Examples of Published Research Priorities in Nursing
B. Examples of Contents from *The Annual Review of Nursing Research*
C. Examples of Research Abstracts
D. Examples of Research Instruments
E. Statistical Software Packages for Microcomputers
F. Sample Patient Consent Form and Information Sheet
G. Excerpts from the American Nurses' Association *Human Rights Guidelines for Nurses*
H. Regional Nursing Research Organizations
I. Sample Query Letter to an Editor
J. Example of a Grant Application

APPENDIX A

Examples of Published Research Priorities in Nursing

RESEARCH PRIORITIES IN GERONTOLOGIC NURSING FOR LONG-TERM CARE* (IN RANK ORDER)

Priorities Extremely Important for Patient Welfare

1. Prevention, formation, and treatment of decubiti.
2. Coping mechanisms needed by the family and patient after discharge.
3. Increase of physician interest in geriatrics.
4. Age differences in response to medications.
5. Improvement in gerontologic preparation of ancillary and nursing students and staff.
6. Epidemiology and treatment of urinary tract infection including catheter care.
7. Common eating patterns and preferences of older adults.
8. Improvement of physician follow-up of patients.
9. Strategies to improve nurse-physician communication.
10. Strategies for attracting and retaining knowledgeable, interested staff.

---

*From Brower, H.T., and Crist, M. (1985). Research priorities in gerontologic nursing for long-term care. *Image*, *17*(1), 22–27.

RESEARCH PRIORITIES FOR CANCER NURSING*

Having the Greatest Impact on Patient Welfare, Ranked from Highest Mean Score to Lowest Mean Score

1. Determine effective methods of relieving chemotherapy or radiation induced nausea and vomiting.
2. Study nursing interventions for the relief of pain in individuals with cancer.
3. Establish discharge planning and follow-up programs which effectively mobilize patient, family, and community resources.
4. Identify nursing interventions which assist patients and families to cope with grief and impending death during the pre-terminal and terminal stages of disease.
5. Find effective ways to prevent and/or treat stomatitis resulting from chemotherapy.
6. Determine most effective techniques for venipuncture, maintenance of intravenous lines, and preservation of veins for patients receiving long-term antibiotic or chemotherapy.
7. Delineate modifications in physical plant, nursing care program, and policy which promote comfort and dignity for the hospitalized terminally ill individual.
8. Establish effective analgesia protocols for patients with cancer.
9. Develop more effective methods of psychological support for patients and families at various stages of disease and cancer treatment.
10. Clarify the dying patient's rights to make decisions about his health care program and establish more effective mechanisms for the exercise of those rights.

---

*From Oberst, M.T. (1978). Priorities in cancer nursing research. *Cancer Nursing, 1*, 285.

RESEARCH PRIORITIES FOR CRITICAL CARE NURSING* (IN RANK ORDER)

1. What are the most effective ways of promoting optimum sleep-rest patterns in the critically ill patient and preventing sleep deprivation?
2. In light of the nursing shortage, especially in critical care nursing, what measures can be taken to prevent or lessen burnout among critical care nurses?
3. What type of orientation program for critical care nurses is most effective in terms of cost, safety, and long-term retention?
4. What effects do verbal and environmental stimuli have on increased intracranial pressure in the head-injured patient?
5. What are the most effective, least anxiety-producing techniques for weaning various types of patients from ventilators?
6. What types of patient classification systems are the most valid, reliable, and sensitive in determining staffing ratios in critical care units?
7. What types of incentives (e.g., wage scales, recognition programs, "clinical ladder," etc.) will retain nurses in critical care units?
8. What are effective ways of reducing staff stress in critical care areas?
9. What are effective nursing interventions in patients with impaired communication (e.g., intubated patients, aphasic patients) to minimize anxiety, helplessness, and pain?
10. What are the effects of patient positioning on cardiovascular and pulmonary functioning of various types of critically ill patients?
11. What are the most effective staffing patterns (e.g., 12-hour shifts, rotating nurses to non-critical care areas) to reduce burnout and provide continuity of patient care?

---

*From Lewandowski, L.A., and Kositsky, A.M. (1983). Research priorities for critical care nursing: A study by the American Association of Critical-Care Nurses. *Heart and Lung*, *12*(1):39.

APPENDIX B

Examples of Contents from *The Annual Review of Nursing Research*

VOLUME 1, 1983

I. Research on Nursing Practice

1. Nursing Research Related to Infants and Young Children — *Kathryn E. Barnard*
2. Nursing Research Related to Schoolaged Children and Adolescents — *Mary J. Denyes*
3. Adulthood: A Promising Focus for Future Research — *Joanne Sabol Stevenson*
4. Clinical Geriatric Nursing Research — *Mary Opal Wolanin*
5. Nursing Research on Death, Dying and Terminal Illness: Development, Present State, and Prospects — *Jeanne Quint Benoliel*

II. Research on Nursing Care Delivery

6. Nursing Staff Turnover, Stress, and Satisfaction: Models, Measures, and Management — *Ada Sue Hinshaw and Jan R. Atwood*
7. Interorganizational Relations Research in Nursing Care Delivery Systems — *Janelle C. Krueger*

III. Research on the Profession of Nursing

8. Socialization and Roles in Nursing — *Mary E. Conway*

IV. Other

9. Philosophic Inquiry — *Rosemary Ellis*

VOLUME 2, 1984

I. Research on Nursing Practice
1. Family Research in Nursing — *Suzanne L. Feetham*
2. Health Promotion and Illness Prevention — *Nola J. Pender*
3. Psychosocial Anxiety in Pregnancy: Relationship to Maternal, Fetal, and Infant Health Status — *Regina P. Lederman*
4. The Experience of Being a Parent — *Angela B. McBride*
5. Coping with Elective Surgery — *Jean E. Johnson*

II. Research on Nursing Care Delivery
6. Assessment of Quality of Nursing Care — *Norma L. Lang and Jacqueline F. Clinton*
7. Public Health Nursing Evaluation, Education, and Professional Issues, 1977–1981 — *Marion E. Highriter*

III. Research on Nursing Education
8. Research on the Teaching-Learning Process in Nursing Education — *Rheba de Tornyay*
9. Nursing Students: Selection, Performance, and Values — *Patricia M. Schwirian*
10. Design and Evaluation of Nursing Curricula: A Critical Review of Research — *Marilyn L. Stember*

IV. Research on the Profession of Nursing
11. Information Processing in Nursing Practice — *Margaret R. Grier*

V. Other
12. Nursing Research and Health Policy Analysis — *Nancy R. Milio*
13. Nursing Research in Canada: A Critical Review — *Margaret C. Cahoon and Margaret Allemang*

APPENDIX C

Examples of Research Abstracts

THE CARDIAC PATIENT AND EXERCISE: A SOCIOBEHAVIORAL ANALYSIS

by Karyn Holm, RN, PhD
Nancy Fink, RN, MS, CCRN
Norma J. Christman, RN, PhD
Norma Reitz, RN
William Ashley, MD

Health beliefs (health motivation, perceptions of severity of illness, perceptions of resusceptibility, efficacy of treatment, barriers to treatment and cues to taking health related action), health locus of control, patient satisfaction, social support, and self-motivation were studied in a group of cardiac patients (N=41; 39M, 2F) who initiated and completed a phase II outpatient cardiac exercise program. Twenty-three were post myocardial infarction (MI) and 18 were post coronary artery bypass graft surgery (CABG). They ranged in age from 34–75 years with a mean of 53.5 years.

In terms of health beliefs, the only subscales not reflecting the tendency toward compliant behavior were general health motivation and cues to taking health related action. Scores on the remaining measures revealed a tendency for subjects to be externally controlled, satisfied with the program and staff, recipients of social support, and self-motivated. Although it was anticipated that MI patients would differ significantly from CABG patients in terms of the measures, this

---

From Holm, K., et al.: The cardiac patient and exercise: A sociobehavioral analysis. *CHART*, *82*(7):13, July 1985. Reprinted by permission of *CHART*, the official publication of the Illinois Nurses Association.

was not found to be true. A correlation matrix revealed that the most remarkable relationships were those between perceptions of severity of illness and general health motivation; health locus of control and general health motivation; perceptions of severity and resusceptibility; and cues to taking health related action and satisfaction with program and program staff. Interestingly, perceptions of resusceptibility were negatively related to social support and self motivation.

The findings provide a basis for future comparisons. The sample possessed characteristics of what others have called the exercise dropout (history of smoking and blue collar worker). They were able, however, to maintain an exercise commitment for a 12-week period. It may be that families and other support systems were instrumental in exercise maintenance as well as health belief factors such as the tendency for both MI and CABG patients: to believe exercise helped their condition, to follow a physician's advice without question, to perceive their condition as serious, and to state that there were few barriers to attending the exercise sessions. Furthermore, the sample's external locus orientation is the antithesis of that traditionally ascribed to the complier. It is therefore suggested that suffering an acute cardiac event may precipitate feelings of externality in those who in other circumstances may be internally controlled.

EVALUATION OF A STRUCTURED DISCHARGE TEACHING PROGRAM ON KNOWLEDGE AND COMPLIANCE IN CORONARY ARTERY BYPASS PATIENTS

Sue Penckofer, RN, MS
Julie Rovtar Marshall, RN, MS
Jane Llewellyn, RN, DNSc

A convenience sample of two comparable groups of bypass patients was studied in order to assess the effectiveness of a structured teaching guide used by nurses in educating the patient and his/her family about normal postoperative recovery. Preoperative health assessments were done on 64 patients and risk factors for heart disease were identified for each individual. One group was educated by an unstructured method; the other group received structured teaching with use of a guide developed by nurses experienced in post open-heart recovery. Knowledge was assessed prior to the institution of teaching and on discharge from the hospital. All patients were again assessed at six weeks post-discharge for postoperative health and compliance with their health risk factors identified earlier. An analysis of variance with repeated measures revealed that both groups had higher total knowledge scores postoperatively. Most postoperative health behaviors (angina, smoking, hypertension, and diet) were comparable between groups. However, those patients who had structured postoperative teaching walked more blocks after surgery ($\bar{x}$ = 15.61) than those patients who received routine teaching ($\bar{x}$ = 7.00) ($p < .005$) although these two groups were not equivalent preoperatively. In addition, the patients who had structured teaching had higher total compliance scores ($\bar{x}$ = 86.8) that those who had unstructured teaching ($\bar{x}$ = 79.5) ($p < .05$). Therefore, although structured teaching may not have initially affected patients' knowledge, it may have had an impact on their compliance with postoperative health behaviors.

From Penckofer, S., et al.: Evaluation of a structured discharge teaching program on knowledge and compliance in coronary artery bypass patients. *CHART*, *82*(2):4, February 1985. Reprinted by permission of *CHART*, the official publication of the Illinois Nurses Association.

APPENDIX D

Examples of Research Instruments

EXAMPLE OF QUESTIONNAIRE TO ELICIT SUBJECT INFORMATION

SUBJECT INFORMATION SHEET

Identification Number ______________________ **Date** ___________

The following information is needed for the statistical analysis of the results of this study. Please respond to the questions to the best of your ability. Circle only one answer for each question. Remember, all information will be kept completely confidential.

1. On an average night, how many hours do you usually sleep? (*Please circle one.*)

   Less than 6 hours in 24 1
   7 to 8 hours in 24 2
   9 or more hours in 24 3

2. Do you currently smoke cigarettes? (*Please circle one.*)

   Yes.......... 1
   No (*If no, skip to question number 4.*).......... 2

3. Do you currently smoke: (*Please circle one.*)

   Less than 1 cigarette per day.......... 1
   Less than ½ pack per day 2
   Between ½ pack and 1 pack per day 3
   More than 1 pack per day 4

4. Do you ever drink alcoholic beverages? (*Please circle one.*)

   Yes.. 1

   No (*If no, skip to question number 6.*).................... 2

5. Do you currently drink: (*Please circle one.*)

   Less than 1 drink per week.................................... 1

   1 to 2 drinks per week 2

   3 to 6 drinks per week 3

   7 to 24 drinks per week.................................... 4

   25 or more drinks per week 5

   (*One drink = 12 ounces beer or 4 ounces wine or 1 ounce liquor*)

6. Do you ever drink beverages containing caffeine, such as coffee, tea, cola drinks, or hot chocolate? (*Please circle one.*)

   Yes.. 1

   No (*If no, skip to question number 8.*).................... 2

7. On the average, about how many caffeine-containing beverages do you drink? (*Please circle one.*)

   Less than one per day 1

   1 to 2 beverages per day 2

   3 to 6 beverages per day 3

   7 or more beverages per day.................................... 4

8. Do you exercise regularly? That is, do you have some sort of exercise program for yourself? (*Please circle one.*)

   Yes.. 1

   No (*If no, skip to question number 11.*) 2

9. How would you classify your personal program of exercise? (*Please circle the* <u>*one*</u> *category that best describes your* <u>*overall*</u> *program.*)

   Light, such as walking, bowling, golf 1

   Moderate, such as dancing, yoga, bicycling, or slow swimming.. 2

   Strenuous, such as running, gymnastics, tennis, swimming 3

Very strenuous, such as cross-country running, basketball, endurance swimming 4

Unsure, specify type ________ 5

10. How often do you usually exercise? (*Please circle one.*)

1 to 2 times per month 1

3 to 4 times per month 2

2 times per week 3

3 or more times per week 4

11. On an average day, about how much walking do you do? (*Please circle one.*)

Equivalent to 5 blocks or less per day 1

Equivalent to 6 to 15 blocks per day 2

Equivalent to 16 to 20 blocks per day 3

Equivalent to more than 20 blocks per day 4

12. To the best of your recollection, when was the start of your last menstrual period? (*Please circle one.*)

4 days or less than 4 days ago 1

5 days to 3 weeks ago 2

More than 3 weeks ago 3

13. Approximately when do you expect your next menstrual period to begin? (*Please circle one.*)

Within the next 4 days 1

Within the next week to 2 weeks 2

Within the next 3 to 4 weeks 3

14. In which clinical department do you work?

Community 1

Gerontology 2

Medicine 3

Obstetrics 4

Pediatrics 5

Psychiatry 6

Surgery 7

15. What is your background?

American Indian	1
Oriental/Asian American	2
Hispanic/Latin American	3
Black/African American	4
White/Caucasian	5
Other, specify ________	6

16. What is your birthdate? ________/________/________
day *month* *year*

This completes the questionnaire. Thank you very much for your responses.

EXAMPLE OF OBSERVATIONAL DATA INSTRUMENT*

XYZ PROJECT

DATA COLLECTION SHEET

Patient Identification Number ___ ___ ___ ___ ___
1 2 3 4 5

Date ___ ___ – ___ ___ – ___ ___
6 7 8 9 10 11

BEHAVIORAL CUES INDEX: While making observations of the patient, indicate the appropriate category of patient behavior.

___
12

Body activation (*Circle one*)

1. Severe anxiety—continual non-purposeful activity such as nervous mannerisms, turning, etc., or sits stiffly and does not move.
2. Mild anxiety—some motions not purposeful, possibly social in origin. Increased activity when specifics of operation or pain mentioned.

*Adapted from Barsevick, A., and Llewellyn, J. G. (1982). A comparison of the anxiety-reducing potential of two techniques of bathing. *Nursing Research*, *31*(1), 24.

3. No anxiety—no unnecessary motions. Gestures purposeful and appropriate to conversation.

____ 13 **Facial expression** (*Circle one*)

1. Severe anxiety—frowning (depression of eyebrows, V-formation between brows); corners of mouth downward. Expressions of this nature through majority of interview.
2. Mild anxiety—signs of both pleasantness and unpleasantness. Occasional facial expressions of anxiety.
3. No anxiety—facial expressions of contentment or pleasantness. No facial expressions of anxiety.

____ 14 **Vocalizations** (*Circle one*)

1. Severe anxiety—expresses strong, unalleviated anxiety. Use of "I don't know," sighing, inappropriate laughter. Use of high-anxiety words (desperate, panicky, terrified).
2. Mild anxiety—few verbal cues of anxiety. Use of words such as: angry, depressed, concerned, uncomfortable, nervous, frightened, shaky, tense, exhausted, fatigued. Expresses concern when specifics of condition are mentioned. Some inappropriate laughter or sighing.
3. No anxiety—no verbal cues of anxiety. Use of nonanxiety words in conversation (calm, cheerful, contented, determined, happy, optimistic, secure, steady).

____ 15 **Content of Conversation** (*Circle one*)

1. High anxiety—expresses numerous concerns, worries, or complaints. Inability to focus on interview.
2. Mild anxiety—occasional or few expressions of concern, worries, or complaints.
3. No anxiety—no expressions of dissatisfaction, and/or expressions of satisfaction or contentment.

EXAMPLE OF QUESTIONNAIRE TO ELICIT DIETARY CALCIUM INTAKE*

Are you following any special diet now?

No 01
Yes 02

(IF YES) What? ______________________________

Are your taking any vitamins/minerals/other supplements?

No 01
Yes 02

If Yes, What? ______________________________
____

How many times a day? ______________________________
For how long? ______________________________
How much a day (dosage)? ______________________________

Are you or have you ever been allergic to milk or milk products?

No 01
Yes 02

How many servings of the following foods do you consume daily?

Food	Serving size	Number of servings	Calcium (mg) per serving
a) Milk	(1 cup = 8 oz.)	________	× 300 = ___
b) Yogurt	(1 cup)	________	× 300 = ___
c) Cheese	(1 slice)	________	× 300 = ___
d) Cottage cheese	(1/2 cup)	________	× 300 = ___
e) Ice cream	(1 cup)	________	× 300 = ___
		Daily calcium intake (DCI):	___

*From Holm, K., Nolan, J., Dan, A., and Kukreja, S. (1985). Physical activity patterns and bone mineral density. Grant proposal submitted to the Division of Nursing, July, 1985.

How many servings of the following foods do you consume weekly?

Food	Serving size	Number of servings	Calcium (mg) per serving
f) Broccoli	(1/2 cup)	______	× 65 = ___
g) Baked beans	(1/2 cup)	______	× 65 = ___
h) Pizza	(1 slice)	______	× 65 = ___
i) Soup (made with milk)	(1 cup)	______	× 65 = ___
j) Sardines	(3 oz.)	______	× 65 = ___
k) Canned salmon	(4 oz.)	______	× 65 = ___
l) Shrimp	(3 oz.)	______	× 65 = ___

Weekly calcium intake (WCI): ___

DCI + (WCI divided by 7) = Average daily calcium intake: ___

APPENDIX E

Statistical Software For Microcomputers

Package Name	Source	Compatible Hardware
Basic Statistical Subroutines Vol. 1	Dynacomp	All computers
Stattest	Dynacomp	All computers
Advanced Statistical Analysis	Radio Shack	TRS-80 Model I/III
Advanced Statpack Version 4.0	Jini Micro-System	Vic 20; Commodore 64
Descriptive Statistics	ComPress	Apple II, IIe; Bell and Howell; Franklin
Statistical	Keller Software	IBM-PC
Crisp	Crunch Software	IBM-PC
Abstat	Anderson-Bell	IBM-PC

APPENDIX F

Sample Patient Consent Form and Information Sheet

PATIENT CONSENT FORM

This sample is intended as a guide to the preparation of a consent form for application to individual research projects. A complete consent form must be submitted with each protocol prior to review by the Human Investigation Committee.

I, ______________________, an adult (or: legal guardian of ______________________, a minor), have been invited to participate in a study of ______________________ under the direction of ______________________, in which I voluntarily consent to participate.

a. The implications of my voluntary participation in this investigation, its nature, duration and purpose, the methods and means by which it is to be conducted, and the inconvenience and hazards which may be expected have been thoroughly explained to me by ______________________.

b. I have read and understand all written materials which have been provided to me further describing the study and its potential risks and benefits to me.

c. I have been given an opportunity to ask any questions I wish concerning this procedure and all such questions have been answered to my complete satisfaction. I understand that my participation in this study can be terminated at any time upon my request without prejudice to my continuing treatment. I also understand that my participation in this study may be terminated at any time if in the opinion of my personal physician or the director of the study this is in my best interest, and that if I have any further questions or problems I should contact the above named director of the study.

d. (If not applicable check [ ]). I certify that, to the best of my knowledge, I am not pregnant at this time. I agree that if I become pregnant during the course of this study I will notify ______________________________, who is directing this study.

____

Volunteer's Signature and Date
(Please type or print name below line)

____

Relationship

I was present during the explanation referred to above, as well as the Volunteer's opportunity for questions, and hereby witness his consent to participate in the study.

____

Witness's Signature and Date
(Please type or print name below line)

(Attach to this form any written explanation of the study which is to be given to each subject.)

PATIENT INFORMATION SHEET

You have been invited to participate in a clinical nursing research study designed to determine the effect of an exercise program to decrease the likelihood that you will get a blood clot in your legs after surgery. You will be instructed how to perform four exercises and asked to do them each hour while you are awake until discharge. The day before you go home you will have a simple test called an IPG (impedance plethysmography). This test will determine if there are any signs of blood clots and will be free of charge to you. An IPG is painless and does not involve exposure to any harmful substances.

Risks and Benefits

There is absolutely no known risk to you and it is believed that exercise will decrease likelihood of the formation of blood clots.

Withdrawal

You may withdraw your consent at any time without affecting your status as a patient.

If you have any further questions about this study, please contact ______________________________ at ______________________________.

Confidentiality

All identifying information will be kept confidential.

I have read and understand the information in this Subject Information Sheet and have received a copy. I have volunteered to participate based on this information.

________________________ NAME ________________________ WITNESS

________________________ DATE

From Voluz, J., Urbanski, P., and Kull, L. Effect of Lower Extremity Exercise on the Incidence of Deep Vein Thrombosis in Total Hip Replacement Patients. Grant proposal submitted to the Arthritis Foundation, August, 1984.

APPENDIX G

Excerpts from the American Nurses' Association *Human Rights Guidelines for Nurses*

HUMAN RIGHTS GUIDELINES

Nursing Activities and Ethical Issues

In health care practice, the need for protection of human rights is of singular importance in any activity that goes beyond the established and accepted practices of the professional group involved or in which the focus is not directed specifically toward meeting the needs of the individual patient or subject. The generation and refinement of scientific knowledge in nursing will involve nurses increasingly in clinical investigations that emphasize furthering knowledge rather than meeting the needs of patients. Nurses, in their roles as practitioners in hospitals and other institutional settings, may find themselves engaged in clinical research developed and implemented by practitioners in nursing or in other fields. Ethical concerns about the potential violations of human rights become crucial when new and untried techniques and procedures are to be used or when the probable outcomes are unknown or doubtful.

When nurses perform activities that are components of clinical research (whether directed by physicians, nurses, or other investigators), the need for protection of human rights must extend to the practitioners who are expected to participate in new and untried

---

From American Nurses' Association (1985). *Human rights guidelines for nurses in clinical and other research.* Kansas City, MO: American Nurses' Association.

practices as well as to the subjects who are recipients of those practices. The concept of informed consent applies not only to subjects *per se* but also to workers who are expected, as part of their daily work, to implement activities that potentially or actually carry risk for others or have uncertain outcomes.

Implementation of these guidelines implies the need for written statements of the conditions of employment and of special expectations for work performance beyond that usually expected of a person occuping the position of nurse. In advance of such employment, nurses need to know if they are expected to provide medicines, treatments, and other procedures as part of double-blind investigations. They need to know in advance if the work requires them to function as data collectors for research in addition to their roles as nurses engaged in the delivery of patient care services. Conditions of employment must also provide the option of not participating in clinical research if the work expectations are not spelled out in advance of employment.

Conditions of employment in settings in which clinical or other research is in progress need to be spelled out in detail for all potential workers. It follows that anyone employed in work that carries the potential of risk to others need to be advised regarding the types of risks involved, the ways of recognizing when risk is present, and the proper actions to take to counteract potentially harmful effects and unnecessary danger.

Protection of Human Rights

The term *human rights* refers to three basic rights mentioned by Sobel in 1979: (a) the right to freedom from intrinsic risk of injury, (b) the right to privacy and dignity, and (c) the right to anonymity.[5]

Right to Freedom from Intrinsic Risk of Injury

In situations in which the nature of the activities or the research design exposes an individual to increased possibility of emotional, social, or physical injury, the degree of risk must be estimated and specified by the principal investigator or designee. The principal investigator predicts the extent of risk to the individual as compared with the potential clinical benefit or humanitarian importance of the knowledge to be gained.

The prospective subject must be given all relevant information before his participation in activities that go beyond the established and accepted procedures necessary for meeting his personal needs. By virtue of their calling, practitioners in the health professions seek to protect individuals under their care from unnecessary physical or mental suffering.

Nurses must be increasingly vigilant in their concern for subjects and patients who by reason of their situations or illness are not able to protect themselves effectively from an externally imposed threat or injury. They must also be sensitive to the possibility of exploitation of captive populations such as students, the poor, patients in institutions, and prisoners.

Right to Privacy and Dignity

Human beings vary in their values and in their judgments about what is considered invasion of privacy and a threat to dignity through demeaning or dehumanizing conditions. The investigator cannot presume to decide for the other person in the matter of privacy and dignity. Consequently, all proposals, investigative instruments, protocols, and techniques to be used in particular activities and research methods must be specified and discussed with the prospective subject and with workers who are expected to participate in the activity as subjects, data collectors, or both.

Right to Anonymity

Safeguards must be developed so that no unanticipated physical, psychological, or social disadvantage accrues to subjects either during the study or as a result of the dissemination of the findings. If subjects agree voluntarily to share certain specific information about themselves that they may or may not choose to divulge to others in a different context, then the investigator must provide assurance that the subjects' anonymity will be protected. Specific prior consent must be obtained whenever the plan of a study or the report of findings will sacrifice subject anonymity or confidentiality.

Special mechanisms for safeguarding confidentiality and protecting the identity of a subject must be developed if the information is not to remain always under the control of the investigator. Potentially demeaning or dehumanizing conditions merit special consideration from both practitioners and investigators inasmuch as these conditions are in many instances difficult to specify and to protect against. Health care practitioners should be aware that violations of human dignity have many potential long-range repercussions when significant values of the individual are involved.

Subjects

Human rights guidelines apply to all individuals involved in the activities described above. When activities are supported either directly or indirectly by the government or other funding sources, these guidelines apply to patients; outpatients; donors of organs, tissues, and services; informants; normal volunteers including students; and volunteers in groups with limited civil freedom. The latter classification refers to prisoners, to residents or clients in institutions for the mentally ill and the mentally retarded, and to persons subject to military discipline, all of whom tend to fall easily into the class of captive audience and population vulnerable to exploitation.

The choice of minors and groups with limited civil freedom as research subjects can be justified in most instances only if benefits will accrue in the future to them or to others in similar situations or classes. Strict standards governing the use of minors and other groups (including the unborn and the dead) lacking the capacity to give informed consent are being established with increasing frequency by various governmental statutes and regulations.

Society's Obligation and the Public Good

In a democratic society the rights of individuals are of necessity counterbalanced by actions and activities designed for the common good of the collective public. Established public health practices such as the immunization of children against diphtheria and pertussis and the chlorination of public water supplies to prevent epidemics of water-born diseases are examples of societal actions in which personal rights gave way to collective rights for the benefit of society as a whole. These and many other public health practices came into being as a result of research seeking ways to treat and control disease.

Advancement of knowledge about health and health-promoting practices is of value to society as a whole. So too is knowledge about client-patient responses and adaptations to potential and actual health problems and about the effects of different nursing interventions on these responses and adaptations. Just as nurses have an obligation to protect the human rights of patients, so do they have an obligation to support the accrual of knowledge that broadens the scientific underpinnings of nursing practice and the delivery of nursing services. Professional responsibility includes a recognition that research by qualified nurse-scientists is a resource in need of support and encouragement.

MECHANISMS FOR PROTECTION OF HUMAN SUBJECTS IN RESEARCH

Assurance: Informed Consent

To safeguard the basic human right of self-determination, consent to participate in research or unusual clinical activities must be obtained from the prospective subject or his legal representative. Free and informed consent requires an explanation of the study and the procedures to be followed and their purposes; a description of physical risk or discomfort, any invasion of privacy, and any threat to dignity; and an explanation of the methods used to protect anonymity an ensure confidentiality. The subject should also receive a description of expected benefits to himself or to the development of new knowledge. In instances in which control groups are used and therapeutic mesures such as drugs are withheld, appropriate alternative procedures that might be advantageous to the subject should be discussed. Also, subjects need to know they are free to discontinue participation in the study at any time without jeopardy.

In addition to making available explicit information, the investigator should offer to discuss and answer additional questions. If subjects are patients of other practitioners, the investigator has an obligation to discuss the proposed study with that practitioner prior to its inception and to negotiate support for its successful completion.

The subject must give consent voluntarily and without being subjected to overt or covert coercion or deception—and only after receiving all of the foregoing information. If the research design requires some degree of concealment of the true purpose or methodology of the study, it must provide for subseqent disclosure of the nature of the concealment and the rationale for incorporating secrecy as part of the procedure.

On some occasions, a research design involves procedures or possible outcomes that may impinge upon the rights of someone related to the subject, such as a spouse or a parent. In such cases, the informed consent of that individual must be obtained. The informed consent of parents or legal guardians must be obtained for investigations that involve minors or individuals judged to be legally incompetent to handle their own affairs. In instances in which these subjects have the capacity to comprehend the implications of the proposed activity, they also should be asked to give their consent. In these cases, their consent supplements rather than supplants the consent of the parent or other legal agent.

Assurance: Institutions and Agencies

There is increasing public support for systematic accountability to ensure that unintentional professional or investigator bias does not overtly or covertly deny individuals their rights. In almost all circumstances, either the professional nurse or the prospective subject is under the aegis of an institution or agency. The agency is responsible for establishing and maintaining procedures to safeguard human rights. To that end, agencies have established IRBs, whose prime responsibility is the safeguarding of the rights of human subjects. Membership on the review committee should be representative of all occupational groups (including professional nurses) whose members are likely to be involved either directly or indirectly in the implementation of the activities or projects undertaken.

In most institutions, the IRB is responsible for initial and continuing review and approval of each activity for which this process is deemed necessary. The review is designed to determine and assure that subjects' rights have been protected; the procedures proposed for obtaining informed consent are adequate; appropriate records are maintained regarding the selection, participation, and protection of subjects; and circumstances that may or do adversely affect the rights or the welfare of individual subjects are reviewed and acted upon appropriately. In addition, for projects supported by government funds, the institution must provide for appropriate professional attention in case the subject suffers physical, psychological, or other injury as a result of participation in the particular activity. Investigators are asked to explain how and when identifying data are to be destroyed and when the study has been completed.

The report of the President's Commission for the Study of Ethical Problems in Medicine and Biomedical and Behavioral Research cautions that IRBs should not be expected to perform monitoring, investigative, or adjudicative functions.[8] Therefore, to assure that there is no conflict with IRB suggestions, clarification of the manner in which the institution plans to provide continuing review of the project is necessary. In some institutions, permission to proceed with the study is given for one year, with approval for subsequent years contingent upon the IRB's review of a yearly progress report by the principal investigator. The commission strongly suggests that institutions implement a mechanism for monitoring research projects if they do not have one. In some hospitals, such mechanisms are contained under quality assurance committees. The IRB should be informed of all problems that develop during the period of the project, even though it should not do the monitoring itself. The commission also recommends that institutions receiving federal research grants and contracts be required to describe to the funding agency their procedures for responding to reports of misconduct and that such procedures be disseminated throughout the institution so that all persons who might be involved in research with human subjects will know which office to contact and what their rights and protections are. The commission emphasizes the importance of professional societies encouraging adherence to scientific norms and compliance with federal regulations.

There are investigational areas in which, by the nature of the data used and the manipulations applied to the data, consent by subjects is not required. These areas include stored data, information, tissue, body fluids, and other materials obtained in the course or routine professional or clinical observations and activities in which data collection does not involve any increased risk to the subject. According to societal values as represented by the federal government, however, use of these items for research, training, and service purposes may present psychological, sociological, or legal risks to the subject or his authorized representative. Determination of whether such risks are involved and whether the use of the materials is within the scope of the original consent is the responsibility of the institution through its established IRB.

In clinical studies that involve hospital or other institutional staff in addition to the research team, special precautions are necessary for safeguarding the human rights of these employees. If the research design requires actions by persons who are not regular members of the research staff (such as nurses assigned to a clinical unit), steps must be taken to ensure that these persons are informed of the procedures and activities expected of them. Responsibility for obtaining informed consent to participate in research belongs to the principal investigator; it must not be delegated to regular employees of the institution for the sake of convenience. So that all members of the institutional staff know that research is in progress, a copy of the patient's signed consent form should be attached to the patient's hospital record.

To monitor the use of both patients and nursing personnel in research and other special activities, a list of all research projects approved by the IRB must be sent routinely to the nursing department and to other departments likely to be involved in implementing the studies. Conversely, to safeguard against the overuse of patients and nursing personnel in research and other special projects and to provide a mechanism for approving research and special activities within departments of nursing, organized nursing services have a responsibility to develop and enforce written policies and guidelines governing these matters, with special attention to protection of the rights of prospective subjects. Guidelines designed to protect human subjects against violation of their rights must incorporate explicit directions for protecting highly vulnerable individuals who have difficulty in providing informed consent. High-risk individuals include but are not limited to those who are illiterate or lack command of the English language (or other primary language), the poor, and others who may not recognize their right to refuse participation without jeopardizing their care or, for some psychosocial, cultural, or other reason (e.g., age or illness) are unable to comprehend instructions or give directions.

Regarding the issue of risk and compensation to the injured, the code of federal regulations under which the IRBs operate does not require that there be no risk involved in research. That would end all research—indeed, all life. Rather, federal regulations consider human subjects to be at risk only when the risks involved are greater than those the subjects would encounter in the course of their normal activities. The crucial issue relates to the degree to which the subjects may be at risk in participating in the research. The President's Commission, after reviewing the issue, stated that there is moral obligation to compensate subjects for injuries caused by research.[9]

Assurance: Professions

Increased use of hospitals and health care facilities for clinical and other research means that practicing nurses are involved increasingly in research activities. Graduate educational opportunities for nurses have produced a corps of nurse researchers who are actively engaged in scientific study. Yet, stereotyped images of nurses and nursing have in some settings obstructed active participation by nurses on institutional committees for review of reseach. The profession of nursing, through its organizations at the national, state, and local levels, has an obligation to publicly support the inclusion of nurses as regular members of institutional review boards and to make this position of the profession known through written statements of policy.

Because nurses in practice encounter many patients whose rights may be unknowingly or inadvertently violated, the profession of nursing, through its national organization, has responsibility for the development of written policies and guidelines governing the rights of human subjects to guide nurses at many different levels of practice in formulating policies and procedures pertaining to these matters in their own jurisdictions. The professional nurse's responsibility for protecting the rights of human subjects requires that mechanisms be established wherby violations or rights can be reported and actions can be taken to countermand them. The profession of nursing, through its organizations at the state level, has responsibility for the development of mechanisms whereby grievances of nurses resulting from the nurses' knowledge of violations of human rights can be reported and redressed.

SUMMARY

In order for nursing to fulfill its professional obligations in a rapidly changing society, each nurse must develop an awareness of the issues and a framework for dealing effectively with emerging human rights problems. Ethical issues frequently involve conflicting values, and in many individual cases ethical standards are not specified in sufficient clarity to allow for unambiguous decision making. As knowledgeable participants in health care practice and research, professional nurses should involve themselves in institutional policy making and in review board activities.

As knowledgeable participants, nurses should also become informed about the various legal parameters affecting practitioner-client relationships. With respect to human rights, legal accountability focuses upon evidence that the professional practitioners or researchers have not failed in carrying out their responsibility by either intentionally or unintentionally withholding relevant information that might have altered the subject's decision regarding participation in investigative activities. Knowledge about the changing scope of nursing responsibility and the emerging ethical issues affecting all practitioners in health care today is necessary for a professional nursing practice that accepts accountability for the protection of human rights of consumers.

References

1. American Nurses' Association. *Code for Nurses with Interpretive Statements.* Kansas City, Mo.: the Association, 1976, 14.
2. *Ibid.*
3. American Nurses' Association. *Guidelines for the Investigative Function of Nurses.* Kansas City, Mo.: the Association, 1981.
4. American Nurses' Association, *Human Rights Guidelines for Nurses in Clinical and Other Research.* Kansas City, Mo.: the Association, 1975.
5. Sobel, Dava. So That Others Can Live. *Omni* 2:3 (1979), 52–58, 114.
6. Scott, D. W. Ethical Issues in Nursing Research: Access to Human Subjects. *Topics in Clinical Nursing* 4:1 (April 1982), 74–83.
7. *Ibid.*
8. Presient's Commission for the Study of Ethical Problems in Medicine and Biomedical and Behavioral Research. *Final Report on Studies of the Ethical and Legal Problems in Medicine and Behavioral Research.* Washington, D.C.: U.S. Government Printing Office, March 1983.
9. *Ibid.*

APPENDIX H

Regional Nursing Research Organizations

Name	*Address*	*Region Covered**
New England Organization for Nursing	55 Chapel Street Newton, Massachusetts 02158	Maine, Vermont, New Hampshire, Massachusetts, Rhode Island, Connecticut
Southern Regional Education Board (SREB)	1340 Spring Street, N.W. Atlanta, Georgia 30309	Maryland, Delaware, West Virginia, Virginia, Kentucky, Tennessee, North Carolina, South Carolina, Arkansas, Texas, Louisiana, Mississippi, Alabama, Georgia, Florida
Midwest Nursing Research Society (MNRS)	P.O. Box 9117 Cincinnati, Ohio 45209	North Dakota, South Dakota, Minnesota, Wisconsin, Michigan, Nebraska, Iowa, Illinois, Indiana, Ohio, Kansas, Missouri, Oklahoma
Western Interstate Commission for Higher Education (WICHE)	P.O. Drawer P Boulder, Colorado 80302	Washington, Idaho, Montana, Oregon, Wyoming, California, Nevada, Utah, Colorado, Arizona, New Mexico

*Note: Not all states are included in regional organizations.

APPENDIX I

Sample Query Letter to an Editor

Dr. Florence S. Downs
Editor, *Nursing Research*
School of Nursing
University of Pennsylvania
420 Service Drive, SX
Philadelphia, Pennsylvania 19104

February 11, 1980

Dear Dr. Downs:

Attached is a summary of a proposed article reporting my recently completed research on bathing as an anxiety reducing technique. The project, supported by a grant from the Chicago Community Trust, involved a comparison of the towel bath technique with the conventional bed bath. Several parameters of patient anxiety were measured. I believe the results of this study will be of interest to a large number of nurses.

Your consideration of my proposal will be appreciated.

Sincerely,

Jane Llewellyn, M.S., R.N.

Attachment

PROPOSED ARTICLE (Attachment to letter)

"Bathing: A Comparison of the Anxiety-Reducing Potential of Two Techniques"

This article reports on the results of a clinical nursing research project comparing the effects on patient anxiety of the towel bath and the conventional bed bath. The 105 patients in the sample were in two groups—those who would be having invasive procedures and those with unrelieved pain. Anxiety was measured using the State-Trait Anxiety Inventory, the Palmar Sweat Index, and the Behavior Cues Index. The results of hypothesis testing will be presented and a discussion of the implications for nursing practice will be included.

Anticipated length: 4,000 to 5,000 words.

APPENDIX J

Example of a Grant Application

American Nurses' Foundation, Inc.

GRANT APPLICATION

I Title Page

1. Title of Proposal

2. Name of Principal Investigator | 3. Dates of Project: From ______ Through ______

4. Institution in which principal investigator is employed or is enrolled (Please indicate if enrolled ☐ yes ☐ no)
   Department or clinical service ______
   College or University or Name of Service Agency ______

5. Social Security Number | 6. Title of position | 7. Degrees

8. Address and phone number of Principal Investigator *(Individual named in Section 2)*
   Home: Business/School:

   Indicate preferred mailing address with an asterisk(*).

9. Please provide licensure number and state in which principal investigator is currently licensed as a registered nurse.

10. Is Principal Investigator experienced in this area of research? ☐ Yes ☐ No

11. List names of all co-investigators.

12. Research on Human Subjects? ☐ YES ☐ NO If YES, project to be reviewed on (date) ______
    Project reviewed and approved on (date) ______

FINANCIAL ARRANGEMENTS

Indicate selection of Option A or B. If Option B is selected, complete Sections 15, 16, and 17.

13. ☐ OPTION A ☐ OPTION B

14. I, the undersigned, certify that the statements are true and complete to the best of my knowledge and accept, as to any grant awarded, the obligation to comply with terms and conditions in effect at the time of the award.

    ______ *Signature of Principal Investigator* ______ *Date*

15. Name and address of institutional affiliation

16. Name, title, address, and phone number of official signing grant application for the affiliated institution.

17. I, the undersigned, certify that the statements are true and complete to the best of my knowledge and accept, as to any grant awarded, the obligation to comply with terms and conditions in effect at the time of the award.

    ______ *Signature of Official* ______ *Date*

Name ______________________________

II Table of Contents/Check List

(Please review as a check list before submitting proposal)

I Title Page

II Table of Contents

III Abstract (250 words maximum)

IV Total Budget and Funding Sources (if applicable)

V ANF Budget

VI Biographical Sketches (use ANF forms only)

1. Principal Investigator
2. Co-investigator(s)
3. Consultants

VII Project Narrative (5 typewritten pages maximum, excluding references)

VIII Appendices

A. Instruments

B. Documentation of Support and Access

C. Documentation of Consultation

D. Documentation of Human Subjects Review

E. Documentation of Tax-exempt Status
(Budget option B only)

F. Advisor's Evaluation
(If the principal investigator is a student)

Name ______________________________

III Abstract
(250 words maximum)

Name ______________________

IV Total Budget and Funding Sources

(Only applicable if budget exceeds $2,500 requested from ANF)

A. What is the total amount needed to complete this project

B. If the amount above exceeds the $2,500 granted by ANF, please provide additional sources and amounts of funding committed to complete the project (include in-kind goods and services committed.)

Name ______________________

V ANF Budget

(This should not exceed $2,500 and must include justification of items requested.)

PERSONNEL	AMOUNT
SUPPLIES	AMOUNT
EQUIPMENT	AMOUNT
TRAVEL	AMOUNT
COMPUTER COSTS	AMOUNT
OTHER EXPENSES (Please specify)	AMOUNT
	TOTAL

Name ________________________________

VI Biographical Sketch

(Give the following information for principal investigator, co-investigator(s) and consultants.) Copy Form as needed

Name	Title

Present Nationality (If non-U.S. citizen, indicate kind of visa and expiration date)

EDUCATION (Begin with baccalaureate training and include postdoctoral)

INSTITUTION AND LOCATION	DEGREE	YEAR CONFERRED	SCIENTIFIC FIELD

Please indicate if currently in an educational program yes ☐ no ☐

MAJOR RESEARCH INTEREST	ROLE IN PROPOSED PROJECT

RESEARCH AND/OR PROFESSIONAL EXPERIENCE (Starting with present position, LIST TRAINING and experience relevant to area of project. List all or most representative publications. List all previously funded research. Do not exceed (2) pages for each individual.)

Name ________________________________

VII Project Narrative

(Add additional pages — but not to exceed five single spaced typewritten pages total, excluding references.)

Name ____________________

VIII Appendices

F - Advisor's Evaluation

All applicant's who are also students must have their faculty advisor complete this portion of their grant application.

Name of Applicant ____________________

Name of Advisor ____________________ Position ____________________

Institution ____________________ Address ____________________

Signature ____________________ Date ____________________

1. Applicant's status: (check all that apply)

☐ Master's student

☐ Doctoral student

☐ Completed required coursework

☐ Completed qualifying examinations

☐ Dissertation only outstanding

☐ Dissertation proposal approved by the committee

2. Status of research project: (check all that apply)

☐ ANF project idea approved by chairperson/advisor

☐ ANF proposal approved by chairperson/advisor

☐ ANF proposal approved by dissertation/advisory committee

☐ Pilot testing completed

☐ Status of data collection, specify ____________________

3. Evaluation of the applicant:

	Exceptional	Upper 5%	Upper 10%	Upper 25%	Upper 50%	No basis for judgement
Knowledge of major field						
Academic knowledge of area upon which study is based						
Technical research knowledge/skills						
Ability to complete independent data analysis						
Demonstrated research ability						
Ability to work independently						
Perserverance toward goals						
Ability to express self in writing						

4. Your written comments about the applicant will be appreciated. Please be as specific as possible abosut the applicant's ability to conduct the research as proposed. Continue on the reverse side if necessary.

Index

Numbers in *italics* refer to illustrations; numbers in **boldface** refer to the glossary; t denotes tabular material.